NURSING REVISION NOTES

PSYCHIATRIC NURSING FOR GENERAL NURSES

By
D. Gukhool SRN, RMN, RCNT, DN, RNT, B.Ed.
and J. R. Johnson SRN, RFN, RMN, RNT, FETC, FRSH.

Merryl Owen.

D1744375

CELTIC
REVISION AIDS

Celtic Revision Aids

30–32 Gray's Inn Road
London WC1X 8JL

© C.E.S.

First Published 1985

Printed and bound in Great Britain by
Cox and Wyman Ltd. Reading

GENERAL EDITOR'S FOREWORD

The nursing revision series is designed for all nurses in training. The notes are suitable for pre-modular study, post-modular revision and examination revision, and will also be of value to learners undertaking ongoing assessment. While being comprehensive in the major areas of both patient condition and nursing care, they are intended to complement, not replace, existing text books. Each book provides information on basic anatomy and physiology, aspects of investigations and nursing care and practice questions and answers are included at the end of each section. The authors have used their experience in nurse education to select important areas of nursing care for inclusion and I am sure that all nurse learners will find the books of continuing value throughout their training.

P.J. Morland
Lecturer
Department of Education
University College Cardiff

AUTHORS' FOREWORD

These notes were written primarily for general nurse learners undertaking psychiatric nursing modules. As a revision aid for hospital and state final examinations, psychiatric nurse learners, too, will find it of use.

Approaches to the care of the mentally ill have undergone recent changes. The 'nursing process' and the concept of 'activities of daily living' may be mentioned, together with the swing away from the 'medical model', whereby patients were treated only for their clinical conditions. Nowadays, a holistic approach is used. Such care requires a study not only of psychiatry but of psychology, sociology, biology, medicine, and a host of other subjects.

Labelling the patient Schizophrenic, or whatever, attunes the nurse to regarding the patient as just that, and she treats him accordingly. In turn, the patient responds to the environment — including the nurse's attitudes. Thus, he may well indeed appear Schizophrenic. The Rosenthal Effect (the self-fulfilling prophecy) must be constantly borne in mind. This is not easy, since it remains obvious that, were it not for a psychiatric *condition*, the patient would not be in hospital, nor in need of care. If we studiously avoid labels and diagnoses we cannot even begin to care.

For the holistic approach to psychiatric nursing, the reader is referred to the many excellent works available in nursing and medical libraries.

The authors have included several self-test questionnaires designed to test the immediately foregoing knowledge.

The format of this book, due to the nature of psychiatric nursing, is different from the other books in the series. No attempt is made to link *each* condition with nursing care/actions in each chapter, but a specific chapter on treatments and nursing care is included after the introduction to the various conditions.

The authors wish to thank Mr M. J. Jones RMN, Cert. Ed., RNT, for his contribution, particularly in chapter 10.

CONTENTS

1 INTRODUCTION TO MENTAL DISORDERS

Modern psychiatry is that branch of medicine which is mainly concerned with the manifestation and treatment of the abnormal functioning of personality which affects either the individual's subjective life or his ability to adapt socially. The term 'mental disorder' includes all forms of mental dysfunction whatever the cause.

The objectives of this section are to:

1. Describe various forms of mental disorders
2. Outline briefly the classification of mental disorders
3. Differentiate the term 'Neurosis' from 'Psychosis'
4. Give a summary of the symptomatology in mental ilness.

Aetiology of Mental Disorders

One of the most fundamental problems that confront psychiatrists today is their inability to be precise about causative factors of mental illness. Psychiatry is such a vast and complex discipline that searching for a precise cause for a particular mental disorder presents the psychiatrists with a challenge. In this text, attempts will be made to provide a simple approach to understanding some of the causes of mental disorder. In mental illness, multiple causation is the general rule.

The aetiology of mental illness can be described using the following terms:

a Predisposing — an inclination toward illness
b Precipitating — a factor which 'tips the balance' into illness
c Intrinsic — residing in the individual
d Extrinsic — environmental

Predisposing causes

Heredity (genetic or congenital)
Specific genes — a number of psychiatric disorders are genetically determined i.e.

a Chromosomal Abnormalities
b Biochemical Abnormalities

Environmental

Environmental factors can be psychological or social. They are insep-
arable since most of the relevant psychological experiences are
ultimately derived mainly from social events. These include:

a Faulty family environment
b Marital difficulties
c Disturbed childhood experiences
d Economic insecurity
e Loss of self-esteem, employment etc.

Precipitating Causes

Physical

a Brain injury — accidents and operations
b Brain disease — tumour, degenerative disorders, infections etc.
c Toxic factors — septicaemia, alcohol, drugs
d Systemic disorders — any forms of bodily illnesses or diseases.

Psychological

The environment in which an individual lives is much more than a
physical world; it entails close interpersonal interaction within the
family group, pressures impose upon the group from outside as well as
the implication of socio-economic and value systems. The psychological factors particularly relate to the critical life periods or life
situations of an individual, for example:

a Adolescence
b Marriage
c Menopause
d Old age
e Bereavement
f Combat
g Major accidents
h Economic loss
i Loss of status, self-esteem etc.

Intrinsic Causes (Residing in the individual)

Although emphasis is placed upon psycho-social factors in our understanding of the causative factors of mental illness, it is important that
intrinsic cases should not be overlooked.

1. Genetic. A number of psychiatric illnesses are genetically determined.
2. Constitutional. Physical constitution is said to be related to mental
illness e.g. a rotund body build to manic depressive disorders, and a
thin (asthenic) build to Schizophrenia.

3. Personality types. These show some correlation to particular mental disorders.
a Hysterical personality
b Schizoid personality
c Obsessional personality
d Cyclothymic personality (mood swinging)
4. Maturation factors. At certain critical stages of human development, changes occur within the individual which may precipitate mental illness e.g.
a Childbirth
b Menarche (onset of menstruation)
c Puberty
d Menopause

Extrinsic causes
Physical. The following may affect the person's mental state by producing changes to the internal environment of the body.
a Infections
b Physical injury
c Intoxication
d Malnutrition
e Avitaminosis.
Psycho-social. These may result in predisposition to mental illness.
a Conflicts (unresolved)
b Psycho-social stress
c Socio-cultural factors
d Loss of status, self-esteem, prestige etc
e Stress in early childhood.

Classification of Mental Disorders

It is suggested that classification of mental disorder may have several positive outcomes. Various attempts have been made to present a logical approach in classifying mental illnesses. The one presented below is based on the W.H.O. international classification, and is possibly less criticised than others and seems to be an acceptable classification which is simple and widely acknowledged.

Differences between Neurosis and Psychosis

Earlier in this chapter, it was stated that psychiatry is not a clear-cut, simplistic discipline. The illness rarely presents itself in a text-book fashion. This is fascinating because it shows that man is a complex social being with individual differences. We all relate to situations in various ways, adapting strategies learnt during development to cope

Classification Table

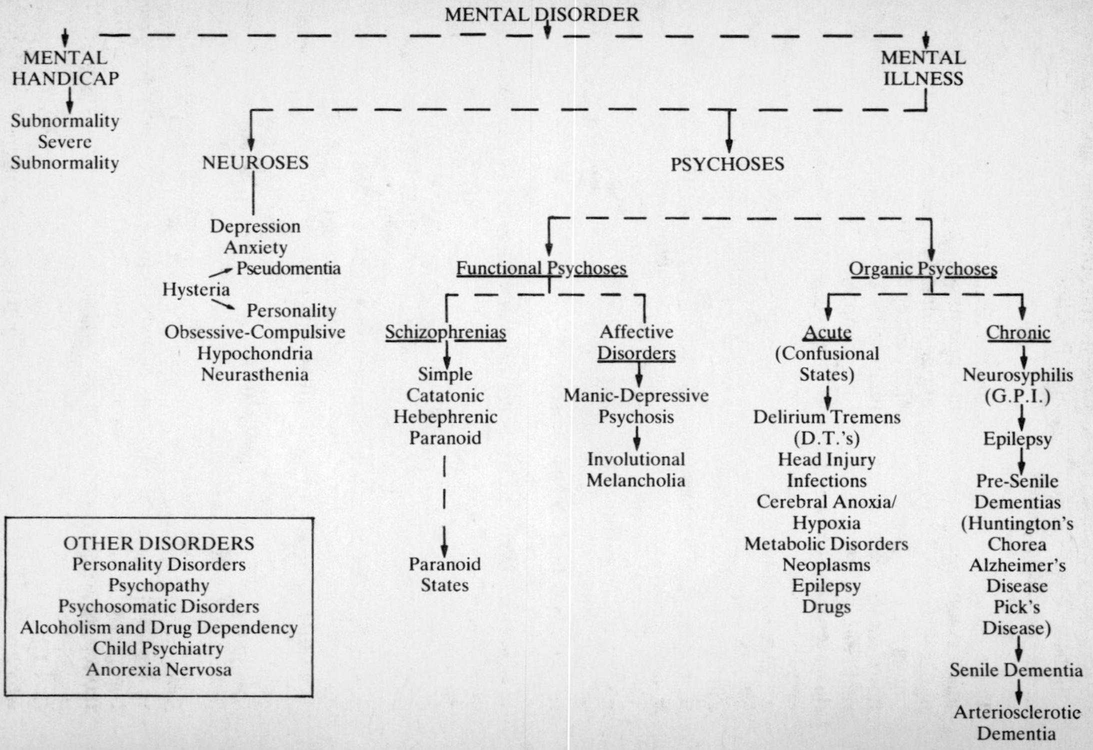

MENTAL DISORDER

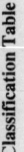

- MENTAL HANDICAP
- MENTAL ILLNESS

MENTAL HANDICAP
- Subnormality
- Severe Subnormality

MENTAL ILLNESS
- NEUROSES
- PSYCHOSES

NEUROSES
- Depression
- Anxiety
- Pseudomentia
- Hysteria
- Personality
- Obsessive-Compulsive
- Hypochondria
- Neurasthenia

PSYCHOSES
- Functional Psychoses
- Organic Psychoses

Functional Psychoses

Schizophrenias
- Simple
- Catatonic
- Hebephrenic
- Paranoid
→ Paranoid States

Affective Disorders
- Manic-Depressive Psychosis
- Involutional Melancholia

Organic Psychoses

Acute (Confusional States)
- Delirium Tremens (D.T.'s)
- Head Injury
- Infections
- Cerebral Anoxia/Hypoxia
- Metabolic Disorders
- Neoplasms
- Epilepsy
- Drugs

Chronic
- Neurosyphilis (G.P.I.)
- Epilepsy
- Pre-Senile Dementias (Huntington's Chorea, Alzheimer's Disease, Pick's Disease)
- Senile Dementia
- Arteriosclerotic Dementia

OTHER DISORDERS
Personality Disorders
Psychopathy
Psychosomatic Disorders
Alcoholism and Drug Dependency
Child Psychiatry
Anorexia Nervosa

with crises in the ways we know best. It is, therefore, difficult to strictly compartmentalise Neurosis and Psychosis without some degree of flexibility and imprecision.

The Neuroses are a group of mental disorders, without any demonstrable organic basis, in which the patients may have considerable insight and unimpaired reality orientation. Behaviour may be greatly affected, but usually remains within socially acceptable boundaries; personality, however, is usually not disorganised — he remains in contact with reality and able to recognise his symptoms. Most neurotics manifest disorders of mood, perception, behaviour, thought and memory. Examples of Neuroses are:

a   Anxiety Neurosis
b   Obsessional Neurosis
c   Depressive Neurosis
d   Hysterical Neurosis
e   Phobias

The psychoses on the other hand embrace two major areas of mental disorders

a   Schizophrenia
b   Manic-depression psychoses.

A summary of the differences between Neurosis and Psychosis

NEUROSIS	PSYCHOSIS
1. Some degree of insight is usually maintained.	No insight in acute cases; insight may improve as patient gets better.
2. Only part of personality is involved.	The whole personality is involved.
3. Over-response to stressful situation.	Flattening of affect (mood) in most situations.
4. Contact with reality maintained.	Patients often live in a fantasy world.

Symptomatology

In the field of mental health as elsewhere in general medicine, we are constantly bombarded with new terminology. Unless we acquire a flavour of the language used in mental health, making sense of this discipline becomes difficult. An attempt is therefore made in this book (See Chap 11) to provide a synopsis of symptomatology in mental illness which will greatly facilitate understanding of various conditions which a nurse may encounter during her psychiatric nursing experience. The synopsis is not for memorisation, but is intended as an initial guide only.

2 SCHIZOPHRENIA

The objective of this chapter is to describe the aetiology, classification and treatment of schizophrenia.

A severe form of functional pyschosis, previously called 'Dementia praecox', (Kraepelin 1896) and renamed 'Schizophrenia' by Bleuler in 1911.

Definition

A related group of mental disorders characterised by dissociation of thought, will, mood, speech and action, and often accompanied by delusions and hallucinations.

Schizophrenia is **not** a 'split mind' in the sense that a dual personality exists, as in the Jekyll and Hyde syndrome. Rather it is a shattered mind, in that psychic functions are disrupted, out of touch with each other and disintegrated.

An analogy

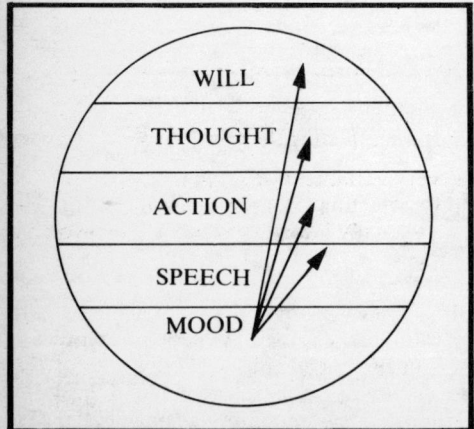

Fig 1 represents a normal mind — individual functions integrated; each affects the others. Hence a depressed mood may lead to reduced will, pessimistic thoughts, reduced action and toneless speech.

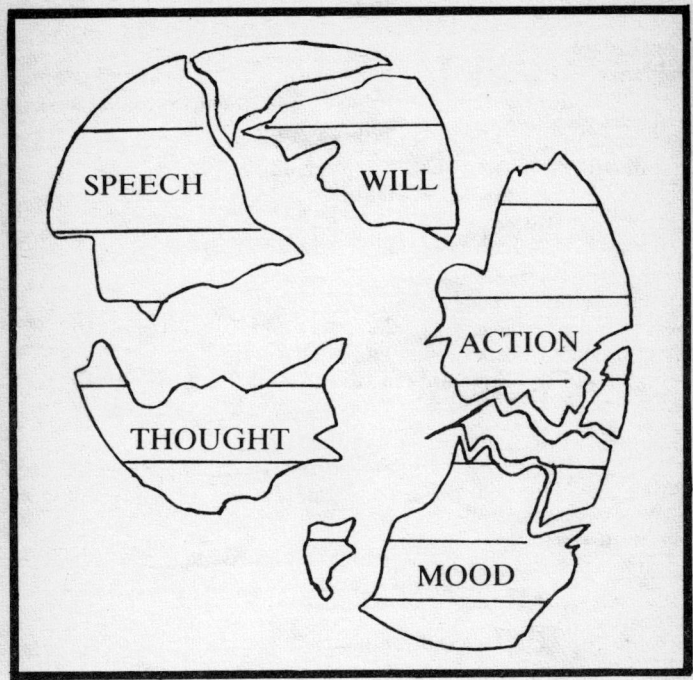

Fig 2 represents Schizophrenia 'The shattered plate' — total disruption. Activities of one part not affecting the others.

The pattern of 'break up' is very variable. For some, the plate shatters into tiny fragments, severely affecting every part of the mind. For others, the plate may remain virtually intact; only a crack or two gives evidence of a breaking-up process.

Incidence
The risk of Schizophrenia is estimated at 0.5 to 1 per cent ($\frac{1}{200}$ to $\frac{1}{100}$).

Also estimated, is that Schizophrenia accounts for 45 per cent of the total hospital population, and certainly constitutes the majority of long-stay patients.

Sex incidence
Somewhat more common in men than in women.

Age incidence
15 years to 25 years commonest onset. Onset later than 40 years is rare.

Symptomatology
A wide variety of signs and symptoms occur, in various combinations. Some of these are found almost exclusively in Schizophrenia and are thus pathognomic. Among the commoner symptoms are found:

Thought disorders — thought blocking, inability to select ideas.
'Knight's-move thinking' — associations between ideas is disrupted.
Pressure of thought/speech/'word salads'.
Concrete thinking — inability to think in abstract terms.
Echolalia — repetition of words and phrases.
Mutism and aphonia.
Neologisms — invented words; a door is a 'swingy jam frame'.
Inappropriate mood responses — laughing at bad news.
Flattening of affect — no mood reactions, mood 'blunting'.
Ideas of reference — neutral things have personal meanings.
Lack of interest in self-appearance.
Lack of motivation, lack of drive, apathy.
Unusual gait and posture.
Withdrawn, cool temperament, social contacts lose importance.
Hallucinations, especially auditory.
Negativism — resistive to suggestion.
Flexibilitas cerea — waxy rigidity, posturing, especially in Catatonia.
Grimacing.
Mannerisms, especially in handwriting.
Delusions — false ideas and beliefs without foundation.

Classification

The subtypes of Schizophrenia are not separate clinical entities, but merely a convenient method of classifying the main features of the condition as they appear in any one patient.

1. Simple Schizophrenia
Onset very slow. Emotional poverty, flattening of affect. Apathy. Social contact withdrawal.

Many of these patients never enter hospital and are content to be tramps, prostitutes and social outcasts.

2. Hebephrenic Schizophrenia
Commonest in late adolescence and young adults. Slow onset. Incongruity of affect. Weird delusions. Severe thought disorder. Giggling, fatuous speech. Childish behaviour.
Named after Hebe — goddess of youth.

3. Catatonic Schizophrenia
Usually acute onset. Severe thought disorder. Stupor, fluctuates with catatonic excitement. Automatic obedience — patient obeys every order without resistance. Flexibilitas cerea — waxy, rigid posturing, often for hours.

4. Paranoid Schizophrenia
Somewhat older patients with fairly slow onset. Fixed delusions of persecutory nature. Thought disorders. Hallucinations.

5. Paraphrenia
A paranoid psychosis of late onset, usually aged 50+. More common in women. Paranoid, narrow outlook, 'chip on shoulder', rigid in attitudes, resentful and with fixed, firm delusions of persecution and of being 'put upon'.

Typically, the deterioration of personality which hallmarks the schizophrenic is absent, and the prognosis is better. Hence, many psychiatrists believe this to be not a form of Schizophrenia, but more related to Manic-Depressive Psychosis.

6. Defect state
This refers to Schizophrenia in its chronic state, often referred to as 'burned-out Schizophrenia'. Many patients in psychiatric hospitals show this condition, together with Institutionalisation.

Negative symptoms predominate. Apathy, lack of drive and ambition. Poverty of thought, blunting of affect. Solitary, withdrawn, aimless.

There is a current vogue to refrain from making a firm diagnosis of Schizophrenia, as this smacks of 'labelling'. Clinical features rapidly shift and what may be Hebephrenic Schizophrenia one day will appear the following day as Simple Schizophrenia. This, however, is no reason to discard the baby with the bathwater. Psychiatric labels are not unchangeable and discarding a name and substituting a 'better' one does not always work, e.g. Madhouse was discarded for Asylum (a better word with its connotations of refuge), but no-one today would dream of calling our Mental Hospitals 'Asylums'.

Classically Schizophrenia is classified into:
1. Simple   — Bleuler 1911
2. Catatonic
3. Paranoid   — Kraepelin 1899
4. Hebephrenic
5. Paraphrenic

Cameron's classification:

(i) Aggressive	Persecuted
	Grandiose
	Self-punitive
	Compliant
(ii) Submissive	Dedicated
	Transformed
(iii) Detached	Avoidant
	Adient

Adience refers to the making of approaches to others. Cameron's classification is interesting but adds little to our knowledge. Simple Schizophrenia seemingly does not exist, whilst Paranoid, Catatonic and Hebephrenic have merely been renamed as Aggressive, Submissive and Detached, respectively.

Schneider, Kleist and Leonhard have each re-classified Schizophrenia according to the presenting signs and symptoms.

Aetiology of Schizophrenia

Cause largely unknown. . . .

Predisposing and precipitating factors obviously important in considering the causes.

a **Heredity** Risk of Schizophrenia in the general public is about 1 per cent. In parents of schizophrenics, 5 per cent. In siblings, 8 per cent, and in children 10 per cent. In identical twins 30–40 per cent.

b **Environment** A 'schizoid environment' possibly accounts for some of the above risk figures. It is probable that a childhood environment provided by affected parents predisposes a child to the disorder if other factors are present.

c **Premorbid personality** The previous personality of the schizophrenic patient was often schizoid; a withdrawn, isolated, unemotional individual of esoteric tastes and interests.

d **Biochemistry** Inconclusive results of research on serotonin and neuro-chemical transmitters. Hallucinogenic drugs e.g. LSD, Mescaline, Psilocybin, known to produce states akin to Schizophrenia. Nitrogen retention is another possible lead; known to be involved in at least one type of schizophreniform illness.

e **Social isolation** Poor areas of cities tend to have both the lowest and highest incidences of social isolation. The relationship with Schizophrenia is noted when patients are most commonly referred from where social isolation is a feature of the environment. Whether this isolation incubates Schizophrenia, schizoid families create such isolation, or whether schizophrenics gravitate to areas of social isolation, is a moot point.

f **Social class** 45 per cent of schizophrenics come from Social Class 5, although Social Class 5 constitutes only 18 per cent of the total population.

g **Physique** The work of Kretschmer, Sheldon and Parnell is well known and all link Schizophrenia with a tendency to an asthenic build and a cerebrotonic personality. However, because of such work, many psychiatrists' diagnoses will be influenced by the patient's physique.

Atypical Schizophrenias

Many states of 'mixed psychosis' occur which do not fall neatly into any one category. Mayer-Gross, Meduna and McCulloch grouped together all schizophrenic complexes where clouding of consciousness is a feature and called them **Oneirophrenia**. Bleuler's '**Latent Schizophrenia**', a variety of undeveloped Schizophrenia in persons of strange distorted personalities, is now considered to be a form of psychopathic personality. Hoch and Polatin described a form of Schizophrenia presenting as a neurosis, and called it **Pseudoneurotic Schizophrenia**. Later work suggests in fact that this is **Neurotic Pseudoschizophrenia**. **Pfropf Schizophrenia** occurs in the mentally handicapped. Whether this is a grafted Schizophrenia on a pre-existing subnormality, or whether it is a mis-diagnosed Schizophrenia of childhood resulting in subnormality is a debated point.

Infantile Schizophrenia
(i)	Heller's	'Dementia infantilis'
(ii)	de Sanctis	'Dementia precocissima'.
(iii)	Kanner's:	'Infantile autism'.

In Heller's disease: normal development for 2-3 years, then advancing schizophreniform complex. Heller stresses bright appearance of these children compared with 'orthodox' mentally subnormal. De Sanctis described children in alternating catatonic excitement and stupor as 'Dementia precocissima' — rare, some say, non-existent. Kanner's disease is the 'Autism' already known, but not labelled schizophrenic as such.

Anorexia Nervosa — a link with Schizophrenia?
Bruch, Mayer and Selvini have all studied A.N. in depth, and agree that it is a schizophreniform disorder.

Selvini, in particular, has shown that the condition is common among those of a pre-existing schizoid personality. A.N. develops almost as a defence mechanism against an imminent slide into frank Schizophrenia. Body and Mind are dissociated and the former is seen as being parasitic upon the Self, and grows, at puberty, at the expense of a fragile mind.

Anorexia means 'without appetite' — a misnomer, since anorexics have a ravenous appetite, but savagely subdue it to 'preserve the identity'. Selvini has used the term 'intropersonal Paranoia' to best describe the phenomenon.

Punishment of the body for sins of the mind was a feature of the Middle Ages where self-flagellation was practised by ascetics. Is Anorexia Nervosa a modern version of self-flagellation? The 'hair-shirt' philosophy is prevalent today.

'If it's unpleasant or difficult, it must be good for you'. Freud had some insight into this when he spoke of a 'death wish'. This view of Anorexia Nervosa may be simplistic, but were the complex psychodynamics of the condition fully known, they would be as utterly baffling as orthodox Schizophrenia, and as curable, i.e., not at all.

Treatment

Phenothiazine drugs are effective when given in comparatively large doses. The most commonly used compound is **Chlorpromazine ('Largactil').** Thought disorders and disturbed behaviour respond well to, for example, 100 mgm three times per day. The affective component of Schizophrenia (emotional blunting, flattening of affect) and the loss of will (as in Catatonia) respond less well. Some psychiatrists advocate concurrent Electroplexy (E.C.T.), particularly where a depressive element exists in the patient.

Long-acting, slow-release drugs, e.g. fluphenazine decanoate, are also widely used, since drug therapy must be continued for years. Such drugs are especially useful for the out-patient, who can attend periodic depot injection clinics, or have the injections given by a Community Psychiatric Nurse in the patient's own home.

An individually tailored programme of social and industrial rehabiliation is required to prevent chronicity. Nurses, Occupational Therapists, Clinical Psychologists, Industrial Therapists, Social Workers and voluntary agencies need to be co-ordinated to provide the necessary care for, if necessary, many years. The programme may well utilise the full resources of the local health services, and involve day care centres, halfway hostels, industrial training units, day hospitals and night hospitals as well as in-patient care in wards of psychiatric hospitals.

1. Practice Questions

Test your knowledge and understanding of the chapter on Schizophrenia by answering the following questions. Avoid referring to the answers until you have answered all questions, then revise from the text those which you answered wrongly.

1. Schizophrenia is:
    a a psychoneurosis
    b a functional psychosis
    c a toxic psychosis
    d an organic psychosis

2. Schizophrenia is characterised by:
    a Disintegration of mental functions
    b Pre-senile dementia
    c Predominantly affective disturbance
    d Clouded consciousness

3. The incidence of Schizophrenia is about:
    a 1 in 70–80
    b 1 in 100–200
    c 1 in 200–300
    d 1 in 300–500

4. Schizophrenia appears to occur more commonly in:
    a Older women
    b Young women
    c Older men
    d Young men

5. 'Pathognomic' means:
    a Serious
    b Diagnostic
    c Sad
    d Invariable

6. The psychiatric term 'Affect' means:
    a Mood
    b Result of
    c False
    d Ingoing

7. Hallucinations are common in Schizophrenia. Usually these are:
    a Visual
    b Tactile
    c Gustatory
    d Auditory

8. Giggling, fatuous speech and childish behaviour are characteristic of:
    a Simple Schizophrenia

b Catatonic Schizophrenia
c Hebephrenic Schizophrenia
d Paranoid Schizophrenia

9. In paraphrenia, deterioration in personality is commonly:
   a Of acute onset
   b Very slow or absent
   c Total
   d Intermittent

10. The defect state of chronic Schizophrenia is often accompanied by:
    a Fits
    b Manic episodes
    c Catalepsy
    d Institutionalisation

11. Which of the following substances is known to produce a schizophreniform condition:
    a Imipramine
    b Mescaline
    c Dopamine
    d Fluphenazine

12. About 45% of schizophrenic patients come from Social Class:
    a 1–2
    b 2–3
    c 3–4
    d 5

2. True or False?

Mark the following statements, True or False.

a Schizophrenia is a split mind.
b The term Schizophrenia was coined by Alfred Adler.
c Adience means avoiding others.
d Clouding of consciousness is a feature of Oneirophrenia.
e In Anorexia Nervosa there is a loss of appetite.
f Pfropf Schizophrenia occurs in the mentally handicapped.
g Schizophrenia most commonly occurs in those of pykno-athletic build.
h Phenothiazine drugs have a dramatic effect upon the affective component of Schizophrenia.
i Electroplexy (E.C.T.) is always contraindicated in Schizophrenia.
j Flexibilitas cerea is a feature of Paranoid Schizophrenia.
k The principal cause of Schizophrenia is still unknown.
l Dementia Praecox is the old name for Schizophrenia.

Answers on page 16.

Answers

1.

1. **b**
2. **a**
3. **b**
4. **d**
5. **b**
6. **a**
7. **d**
8. **c**
9. **b**
10. **d**
11. **b**
12. **d**

2.

a. False
b False
c False
d True
e False
f True
g False
h False
i False
j False
k True
l True

3 AFFECTIVE DISORDERS

The objectives of this chapter are:
a   To describe the commoner forms of depression and mania.
b   To state some of the known causes.
c   To outline the treatments available.
d   To present the salient points about suicide.

We are all aware of having felt depressed at times. Perhaps these minor depressions result from some external factor, e.g. a bereavement or merely a 'Monday morning feeling'. At other times, we may get an attack of the 'miseries' for no known reason. The former we could call **exogenous** (or **reactive**) depression, and the latter we call **endogenous** depression.

On occasions, too, we may feel quite elated and 'everything in the garden is lovely'. And we all know at least someone who seems permanently 'high' and jolly.

These mood (affect) variations are generally of a very minor nature and certainly do not require treatment. We know that our upswings and downswings of mood are only temporary. In this respect such mood variations can be called subclinical and self-limiting.

Imagine now an attack of the miseries multiplied by ten, and you have some conception of how a patient feels when suffering from **Clinical Depression**. Then imagine your mild elations multiplied by ten, and you have a conception of **Mania**. You find it hard to imagine? Not surprising; we often think we know what clinical depression is like, but would be appalled at the severity if we really suffered from it.

Clinical Depression

The depressed mood may arise 'out of the blue', for no obvious reason — called **Endogenous** or **Psychotic** Depression, or it may be an extended severe reaction to depressing circumstances — called **Exogenous** or **Neurotic** Depression. When depression only occurs, with no upswings into mania, we talk of the disorder being **Unipolar**. If the mood swings from depression to elation (mania), we talk of a **Bipolar** condition.

The disorder may be **Primary**, i.e., there is no other condition associated with it, or it may be **Secondary** to some other condition, e.g. physical illness or Schizophrenia.

Clinical Picture

In **Endogenous** depression, the patient appears sad, tired, lacking in interest and miserable. His home, social and work activities are much reduced. This is evident enough in a mild case; in a severe case it amounts to a complete cessation of all activity — depressive stupor. The outlook appears to be hopeless to these patients, with nothing but gloom and despondency in the future.

When the depression is accompanied by **anxiety** — which is common — the patient is agitated, restless, wringing hands and endlessly pacing up and down. He may try to control this anxiety by putting on a brave face, the so-called 'smiling depression'.

Depressed patients often show **retardation**, or slowing of thinking and speech. Movements are slow, **as are other bodily activities**, hence constipation, loss of appetite, amenorrhoea, loss of weight and hypotension. Loss of sex-drive (libido) is common.

Feelings of guilt lead to remorse and self-reproach. The patient may think that his condition is a judgement upon him for past sins, and that other people despise him for his wickedness. Totally immersed in his misery, the patient may well have hypochondriacal ideas that may amount to **delusions** (false beliefs) of poverty and bodily disease.

All these signs and symptoms are typically worse in the morning, less severe in the evening (diurnal variation). The patient's sleeping pattern is disturbed too, with no difficulty in sleeping during the evening, but waking very early (say 3.00 a.m.) in acute distress and unable to sleep again. Contrast this with the patient in an anxiety state who typicaly cannot sleep late at night, but sleeps heavily in the morning when it is time for work.

Many patients do not readily admit to feelings of depression, preferring instead to attend their G.P.'s surgery complaining of one or more of the **physical** components of depression only: anorexia, weight loss, amenorrhoea, etc. In the same way that Hysteria and Syphilis are great mimics, depression, too, may present in a dozen different physical disguises. The wise G.P., the wise nurse, looks beyond the immediately obvious. . . .

Exogenous (reactive) depression is much more common than Psychotic Depression. The symptoms are less severe and classically date from a depressing event. The diurnal variation and sleep disturbance of Psychotic Depression are much rarer. On investigation it is frequently found that there are other neurotic tendencies in the patient's personality. Physical treatments such as E.C.T. and chemotherapy are far less effective, and the patient requires treatment for his underlying neurosis, i.e. psychotherapy. In the short term he responds quite well to attention, company, diversional activities and reassurance.

Causes

Sex Incidence. Women suffer from affective disorders more than men; the incidence is about twice that of men. The puerperium and menopause are particularly difficult times and the depressions associated with these events can be very severe. Amenorrhoea is common in depression, and the pre-menstrual distress syndrome is well-known. The suggestion then that there is an endocrine component in depression is well-founded.

Physique. There is a strong association between affective disorders and a pyknik body build, i.e., round face, chubby, short neck and plump.

Age. The incidence rises with age.

Season. Spring and early summer are classically the seasons of mood swings.

Genetics. The general incidence of affective disorders in the general population is largely unknown. Depression tends to be self-limiting, and perhaps the majority of people with transient depressive episodes never reach medical records and statistics. The incidence of manic depressive psychosis is about 1 per cent of the population. In monozygotic (identical) twins the concordance rate is 70 per cent, and in dizygotic (non-identical) twins 20 per cent. In families generally the rate is 10–25 per cent.

Race. Jews and the Irish appear to be more at risk from these disorders than others.

Pre-Morbid personality. There is a definite depressive personality type: gloomy, morbid and lacking in drive. Also there are cyclothymic personalities whose mild mood swings can be accentuated to a pathological degree, and result in manic-depressive psychosis. Kretschmer and Sheldon have shown the link between cyclothymia and the round 'Mr Pickwick' physique mentioned above.

Stress. The link between depression and stressful events is often misleading and questionable. Patients blame their depression upon an event or series of events, but on investigation it is commonly found that the illness pre-dates those events. In times of acute national stress, as in the 1939–45 war, with food rationing, bombing, black-out and family separation (evacuation, and menfolk conscripted into the armed services), the incidence of mental illness, particularly affective illness, declined sharply. Stress, then, appears to be an easy excuse for depression; it is rarely a reason.

Social Isolation. Insecurity and social isolation with loneliness probably account for a great deal of depression.

Drugs. Certain drugs are known to cause depression, notably Reserpine, Phenobarbitone, Methyldopa, Benzhexol and contraceptive pills with a high progesterone content.

Physiological events. Childbirth, the puerperium, menopause, acute febrile or painful illnesses and jaundice may be mentioned as being often implicated.

Mania

Mania is ten times less common than depression and is never chronic. It may exist as an entity in its own right, arising and subsiding spontaneously, or it may occur associated with intermittent depression—manic depressive psychosis.

Mania usually arises in a hypomanic personality with a mild degree of mania not requiring treatment until the disorder progresses to the state where mania or acute mania (Bell's mania) occur. The patient is usually referred for treatment by his relatives, since the patient himself has no insight (does not realise he is ill), and feels perfectly well and happy.

In mania the patient shows cheerfulness, jollity, euphoria and hilarity. Infectious jollity best describes his condition, as his sense of well-being is easily transmitted to those around him — for a while. Over longer periods this sustained jollity becomes tiresome. Flashes of irritability occur, particularly if someone disagrees with the patient.

Mental and physical activity increase, there is sleeplessness and over-talkativeness. The patient's plans for the future are wildly optimistic and well beyond his means. Disinhibited actions and promiscuity may lead to trouble with the police, and his family may suffer from his profligacy, by his spending large sums of borrowed money on whims.

His energy is boundless, but he rarely completes any task, since his attention flits rapidly from one thing to another. Overdressing is commonplace. No one is in any danger of overlooking him at a party, and spontaneously arranged parties are common, the patient inviting large numbers of friends and strangers home, to his family's despair.

The patient's thinking is rapid, even torrential, and his speech follows suit. Rhymes, puns and 'jokey' speech are common.

Delusions are not common, but paranoid ideas are, especially if others frustrate his grandiose plans.

He is often voraciously hungry, but he rarely gains weight, partly because his food intake, though large, does not keep pace with his energy output, and partly because his meals are interrupted and seldom finished, as his attention shifts to things yet to be done. The failure to gain weight is often surprising, since commonly his intake of alcohol is excessive too.

Mania usually lasts from 6–8 weeks, then either subsides, or swings abruptly to depression.

Treatment of Mania
1. Admission to hospital is imperative.
2. Sedatives are used initially to suppress the wild excitement.
3. Tranquillisers, e.g. Chlorpromazine 200 mg 4 times per day.
4. E.C.T.(Electro-convulsive therapy).
5. Lithium carbonate by injection 300–600 mg 3 times per day, reducing to a lower maintenance dose. This drug has many side effects, and since blood lithium levels need to be accurately monitored is suitable only for in-patients, rarely for out-patients.
6. Dietary correction and vitamin supplements.

Treatment of Depression
1. E.C.T (Electro-convulsive therapy), either bilateral, or unilateral to the non-dominant lobe of the brain, is very useful for relieving endogenous depression, but is not effective in treating exogenous (neurotic) depression.
2. Anti-depressive drugs: generally the tricyclic drugs and monoamine exidase inhibitors.
3. Supportive psychotherapy.
4. Occupational and diversional therapy.
5. Social reintegration.

Prognosis
This is variable in affective conditions, but the chemotherapy usually prescribed, e.g. Imipramine, can maintain the patient in the community for long periods.

Suicide

Suicide and attempted suicide (parasuicide) are perhaps commoner than most people (even nurses) realise. The general nurse, working in a casualty unit, may well have more insight into its prevalence than the psychiatric nurse, but even she — the general nurse — rarely appreciates the size of the problem.

Every minute and a half a suicidal death occurs somewhere in the world. In Britain one such death occurs every 8 hours, night and day. Attempted suicide is a least 10 times as common.

Self-poisoning results in 15 per cent of all admissions to medical wards, and in patients under the age of 40 is the commonest reason for admission to those same medical wards.

The myths which surround the subject are many; perhaps the commonest being that those who threaten suicide never do so. Another is that all attempted suicides are hysterical and attention-seeking. These myths are quite untrue, as is the myth that all suicides are mentally ill.

The facts are that suicides tend to be over 45, men, of higher social class and use violent methods. Attempted suicides tend to be under 45, women, of lower social class and use self-poisoning rather than violence.

The Suicide Group
Older men who are single or divorced and socially isolated are those mainly at risk. Redundancy and retirement from (especially) responsible professional jobs add to the risk. A history of bereavement, physical illness or alcoholism is a common feature. Cities, with their paradox of the highest incidence of social isolation, produce more suicides than rural areas.

Death at the first attempt, without warning, is common among men with stable, intelligent personalities; precipitated by the death of a wife. A minority will successfully commit suicide after one or two previous attempts. A history of a disordered personality is common, and talk of suicide usually precedes the attempt. This sub-group is more like the group of parasuicides than the foregoing sub-group.

Attempted Suicide (Parasuicide) Group
The incidence of half-hearted attempts at suicide is higher in younger women, and occurs most commonly as an impulsive reaction to stress. A history of personality disorder is common; immature or anti-social. Alcoholism and drug-taking are frequently implicated. Violence is usually avoided; an overdose of drugs is the usual means.

There are many motives for attempted suicide. For some it is an immature method of 'getting back' at parents or a boyfriend whose interest is waning. 'I'll kill myself, then won't they be sorry . . .?' For a few it may well be a 'cry for help', but for the many it is more a distaste for oneself brought on by a neurotic form of depression.

These patients should not be confused with those genuine accidental overdose cases who misread an instruction on a bottle of tablets. There are cases, too, where having taken a prescribed dose of a sedative to go to sleep, the person wakes, and in a confused sleepy state forgets their previous dose and takes another 'just in case'.

25 per cent of parasuicides will make at least one further attempt at suicide, and some 10 per cent will be successful.

Management and Care

The distress and remorse of a patient waking up in a medical ward, or worse still, a psychiatric ward, after an attempted suicide are not helped by nurses and doctors who are brusque, dismissive and critical. Sympathy, and a genuine wish to understand and help, are the hallmarks of the emotionally mature and experienced nurse. Such a nurse has sufficient insight to realise the extent of the distress the patient must have felt in wishing to destroy herself.

After the initial medical or casualty treatment (gastric lavage, suturing of wounds, etc.) the patient is usually referred to a psychiatrist for assessment of future suicidal risk. Many factors have to be taken into consideration in assessing this risk, among which are:

Previous suidical attempts
Depression
Alcoholism or drug addiction
Family history
Psychopathic disorder
Epilepsy
Bereavement/divorce
Chronic illness
Availability of lethal drugs
Poor housing
Loss of financial and social status
Immigrant

Commonly, all the signs and symptoms of acute depression are present when the psychiatrist sees the patient, and transfer to a local psychiatric hospital is indicated.

Preventing Suicide

Voluntary organisations (Samaritans, etc.) do sterling work in crisis situations. They, and the patient's general practitioner are in the front line of prevention.

On a larger scale, public education and social change are required. Domestic medicine cupboards should be cleared out regularly. Large routine prescriptions are to be avoided in prescribing for any patient.

The reduction of alcoholism and drug abuse in society is more difficult and costly, but is life-saving on a large scale.

Practice Questions

1. Give another name for Exogenous Depression.
2. What is Retardation?
3. What is a Delusion?
4. What is the 'diurnal variation' in depression?
5. Which is the commoner, Reactive or Endogenous Depression?
6. In which form of depression is E.C.T. more effective?
7. What does Cyclothymia mean?
8. To what extent would you say that stress is a cause of mental illness?
9. What is Bell's mania?
10. What is the incidence of suicide in Britain?
11. What general differences exist between men and women in the methods chosen for suicide?
12. What is the other name for attempted suicide?
13. What is the incidence of further suicidal attempts among those who attempt it for the first time?
14. Why is this section on Suicide included under the general chapter heading of Affective Disorders?
15. In Manic-Depressive Psychosis the condition is:
    a Unipolar
    b Bipolar
    c Exogenous, or
    d Reactive
16. Affective disorders are more common in people whose physique is:
    a Pyknik
    b Athletic
    c Asthenic
    d Dysplastic
17. The incidence of Manic-Depressive Psychosis in the general population is about:
    a 0.05%
    b 1%
    c 2%
    d 3%
18. Mania usually lasts:
    a for a few hours
    b for a few days
    c for a few weeks
    d for a few years

Answers on page 26.

Answers

1. Reactive or Neurotic Depression
2. Slowing of thinking or speech, often accompanied by slowing of physical functions, e.g. constipation.
3. A delusion is a false belief or idea, not consistent with the facts and generally unreasonable.
4. Typically the depressed patient feels worst in the morning but improves during the day.
5. Reactive depression is much commoner than Endogenous (Psychotic) depression.
6. In Psychotic depression.
7. Mood swinging.
8. Stress is rarely implicated as a cause of mental illness, though it is often blamed.
9. Bell's mania is the most acute form of the condition.
10. 3 suicidal deaths per 24 hours, and 30–40 attempted suicides in the same period.
11. Generally, men choose violent methods, women choose overdoses of drugs.
12. Parasuicide.
13. 25% will try again.
14. Because suicide is perhaps the most serious complication of depression.
15. In Manic-Depressive Psychosis the condition is bipolar.
16. Pyknik.
17. 1%.
18. For a few weeks; usually 6–8.

4 ORGANIC PSYCHOSIS

The aim of this chapter is to acquaint the general nurse with the commoner forms of psychiatric disorder arising principally from **physical** causes. Included is a section on epilepsy, since this may have a definite organic cause, though in another form it is idiopathic. The objectives are:

a To present the general features of organic psychoses.

b To show how pregnancy and childbirth may be accompanied by psychiatric disturbance.

c To describe Huntington's Chorea as a type of organic psychosis in one of its severest forms.

d To outline what the nurse needs to know about Epilepsy.

e To note some forms of pre-senile dementia.

f To present the psychiatric manifestations of arteriopathic diseases.

g To introduce the subject of old age, which results, in a minority of cases, in senile dementia. This subject is covered more fully in other books in this series.

Two Main Groups

1. Acute psychoses; delirium or toxi-confusional states.
2. Chronic psychoses; once diagnosed are labelled according to the underlying disease, e.g. pre-senile dementia, arteriosclerotic dementia.

The main difference between the two groups is that in the acute syndrome, the symptoms are usually reversible if the underlying disorder is corrected, while in the latter group the pathological changes bring about permanent damage to the central nervous system.

The end result of such damage is dementia. This term only applies to conditions characterised by progressive irreversible damage to brain tissue and function. It should be added that not all acute conditions have a satisfactory outcome as chronic states may have an acute onset.

Features

All organic psychoses affect all mental processes especially:

1. Cognition   — Perception — illusions and hallucinations
                   Thinking   — marked defect of conceptive thinking.
                   Remembering — registration, retention, recall.

2. Mood — Irritability, anxiety — fear. Depression, apathy, euphoria, excitement.
3. Behaviour — This depends on 1. and 2. and on the personality of the patient.

Actual clinical picture varies from patient to patient and on the pathological process.

Acute Organic Psychosis
This is a toxi-confusional state — delirium.

Features
1. Varying degrees of clouding of consciousness plus disorientation.
2. Poor attention — distractability.
3. Perceptual disorders — illusions and hallucinations.
4. Mood of unease to frank terror.
5. Abnormal thinking.
6. Misidentification of people.
7. Symptoms worse with darkness. Drowsy by day and awake at night.
8. Poor recollection of the disorder.

Causes
1. Systemic infections — pneumonia, influenza, typhoid etc.
2. Inflammations and infections of C.N.S. — meningitis, encephalitis.
3. Head injury. Raised intra-cranial pressure. Dementia. Epilepsy. Cerebral tumor.
4. Drugs. Barbiturates. Amphetamines. Hashish. Alcohol. Antidepressants, especially in the elderly.
5. Cerebral Anoxia — heart failure, cerebrovascular disease, anaemia.
6. Metabolic and endocrine — uraemia. Liver failure. Hypoglycaemia.

Children and old people become delirious much easier.

Treatment
a Of primary disease
b Good nursing care — quiet, rest, fluids, adequate sleep.
c Tranquillisers.

Dementia
Main features
1. Memory loss.
2. Impaired judgement and reasoning.

3. Emotional defects — anxiety, irritability, impulsive conduct, alcoholic excess, sexual aberrations.
4. Disorientation, especially at night.
5. Delusions — outcome of faulty perception and judgement.
6. Reduction of personal care.
7. Physical concomitants.

In old age the normal ageing process involves reduced mental and physical capacity, with inability to cope with new situations. There is a tendency to become rigid and fixed. Memory is impaired. There is loss of interest and a tendency to dwell in the past.

Causes of Dementia
1. Senile Dementia — in which there is cerebral atrophy.
2. Huntington's Chorea.
3. Pre-senile Dementia — onset in 50s to 60s.
4. Arteriosclerotic Dementia — a fluctuating disorder with often a history of strokes and focal neurological signs.
5. G.P.I. — (Cerebral syphilis is quite rare in Britain now).
6. Cerebral tumours, especially frontal lobe tumour.
7. Metabolic and endocrine disorders.

Treatment
1. Treatment of the underlying cause may prevent progression of symptoms. The vast majority either have senile dementia or cerebrovascular disease.
2. Good nursing care.
3. Medication — tranquillisers to control disturbed behaviour.

Puerperal Psychosis

This is a rather vague term — how long is the puerperium, and are all such cases psychotic? The answers are 'who knows?' and 'no' respectively.

Puerperal psychosis may occur at any time towards the end of pregnancy and up to three months afterwards. Many cases will present as a frank neurosis, rather than psychosis.

3 people are at risk: **a** the mother
b the child
c the father

The mother suffers the main condition; the child suffers from maternal deprivation, and possibly, infanticide; the father may (rarely) suffer from 'Folie a deux'.

Incidence	2 per 100 births (live births or still births)
Distribution	More common in Western society
Onset	Rather sudden. 2–3 days common
Signs and Symptoms	These vary very considerably, depending upon the patient's previous personality and what predisposing factors are present.

Puerperal psychosis may take the form of **any** psychiatric disorder, ranging from a severe depressive illness to a full-blown Schizophrenic reaction.

More than 50% of all patients have a previous history of mental disorder, and perhaps 90% of the remainder have a rather hysterical personality.

It is not uncommon for women to suffer a depressive phase during the last three months of pregnancy, and if this patient had a previous similar phase during the first three months of pregnancy, she must be suspect of being a likely candidate for Puerperal Psychosis after the birth of her child.

Mild depression within 1 or 2 weeks of childbirth is common — this is to be expected and is a true reactive depression. This does not require treatment, other than support and reassurance.

In 2 cases out of 1,000, the combination of hormonal change and psychological stress will precipitate a severe mental illness of quite sudden onset.

The 2 most common forms of this Puerperal Psychosis are:

Severe Psychotic Depression and Schizophrenia.

1. Depressive type
A patient in acute mental distress, with continual misery, especially in the morning. Wakes early (4 or 5 a.m.) and cannot sleep again. Delusions of unworthiness are common. Crying and moaning, she may be underactive and just sit around neglecting herself and everything else. Or this weeping woman may be overactive, wandering about wringing her hands and in an obvious anxiety state.
N.B. 'Anxiety' in psychiatry **does not mean worry**, it means fear.

In depression there is a serious risk of suicide. Since the woman will see the world as depressing and colourless, she will often commit infanticide before suicide. Separation of mother and child is not however necessary if both are hospitalized at an early stage. Any delay, however, and separation is imperative,
a because the child is in danger of infanticide, and

b because the child will be neglected.

Treatment
E.C.T. (Electro-convulsive therapy) is the fastest method of resolving depression. One session each day for 6 days will usually suffice. Unilateral modified E.C.T. is the method of choice. Alternatively, or conjointly, a tricyclic anti-depressive, e.g. Imipramine (Tofranil) 25 mg twice per day may be used. Even before the birth of the child E.C.T. may safely be used, and is the treatment of choice. Weaning the child and suppression of lactation with oestrogens is usually very advisable.

2. Schizophrenic type
This is somewhat more common than the depressive type, and is more liable to recur with subsequent children. The clinical picture is that of an acute Schizophrenic episode together with an impairment in the state of consciousness.

A working definition of Schizophrenia:

'A group of mental disorders characterised by dissociation of thought, feeling, will, speech and action and often accompanied by delusions and hallucinations.'
There are 4 main types:
Simple Schizophrenia
Paranoid Schizophrenia
Catatonic Schizophrenia
Hebephrenic Schizophrenia

1. Simple Schizophrenia
Most common type. Sudden dissolution of the integrity of the personality. Thoughts, will, moods, speech and action are at variance, to a greater or lesser extent. A vacant wandering, drifting, isolated, indifferent person results. She has feelings of passivity, i.e. feels that her thoughts and actions are being controlled by others. She shows 'incongruity of affect', i.e. her mood is at variance with events. She often appears in a dream-like vacuous state, talking to her 'voices'. Auditory hallucinations are common, but visual hallucinations are rare.
N.B. There is danger to the child. The mother may kill the child because 'God told her to do so'.

2. Catatonic Schizophrenia
Much the same as Simple Schizophrenia, but the will is severely affected. Loss of will and consequent inertia may be fairly mild to severe. Indeed, complete stupor is not uncommon. Interspersed with

brief periods of wild behaviour (Catatonic excitement), she spends long periods inert and unresponsive. 'Flexibilitas Cerea' — a sort of waxy flexibility is a feature of this condition.

3. Paranoid Schizophrenia
As in Simple Schizophrenia. Marked by fixed delusion of persecution and vivid persecutory hallucinations.

4. Hebephrenic Schizophrenia
As in Simple Schizophrenia again, but marked by a childlike pattern of thoughts and actions. Emotional lability is common, with weeping and laughing, silly giggling. Fatuous grinning and posturing are common, and the woman is wholly irresponsible.

In all types, the child is at risk and the mother must not be entrusted with the child.

Hospitalization is usually imperative.

Treatment
Large doses of major tranquillisers, e.g. Chlorpromazine (Largactil) 300 mgm 3 times per day. E.C.T. is used for catatonic stupor.

Prognosis
Good in acute phase. However, since the basic personality is already unstable, attacks are liable to recur. Treatment is usually prolonged (as an out-patient) and further pregnancies should be terminated for 3 reasons:

1. The child is at risk from neglect and infanticide.
2. The mother's mental well-being.
3. Children born of Schizophrenic mothers are liable to develop autism or later Schizophrenia.

Folie a Deux
Used to be called 'Communicated Insanity'. People who have very close emotional ties with the mother, e.g. husband, children, may show evidence of a temporary disturbance resembling the mother's.
N.B. A Schizophrenic father may well cause Folie a Deux in his wife especially in times of stress, e.g. the puerperium. In seeing a case of reported Puerperal Psychosis, always ask yourself: 'Who is the patient?'. Folie a Deux resolves itself without treatment as soon as the real patient has been removed.

Lastly, very common is a mixed Depressive/Schizophrenic type illness in Puerperal Psychosis which resembles a Toxic Psychosis. The hallmark of this condition is the fluctuating state of consciousness. Do not miss it!

Huntington's Chorea

One of the most devastating conditions, physically as well as psychiatrically, is Huntington's Chorea. It is a degenerative disease of the nervous system, running persistently through affected families, and is hereditary. Classically, it occurs in adult life (35 to 40 years) but may occur earlier, and is characterised by progressively worsening choreiform movements of the whole body and by mental deterioration.

Large muscle groups are involved resulting in the typical athetoid writhing movements of the limbs and trunk. These movements are wholly involuntary. The age of the patient is usually sufficient to differentiate this from Sydenham's Chorea (St. Vitus Dance), allied to rheumatism, and affecting children. Progressing from an early nervous fidget, or foot tapping, the involunatary movements become coarse and bizarre, eventually becoming impossibly grotesque. In later stages the movements decrease, and total rigidity supervenes with rapid muscle wasting.

Mentally, the earliest signs are of irritability, emotional lability, violent temper, sexual assault and destructiveness. Psychotic episodes may follow, resembling mania, depressive psychosis or hebephrenia. Feelings of unworthiness and self-reproach lead commonly to suicide, especially if the patient retains insight into the progressive and fatal nature of his disease. Dementia occurs after a few years and heralds death.

Prevalance
Greater than 25 per 100,000 dependant somewhat on geographical area.

Social
Devastating, especially for the spouse and children.

Genetics
Caused by a dominant gene of persistence and penetrance.

Course
The disease on average runs a 15 year course with death at 55 years.

Statistically
There is a $^{50}/_{50}$ chance of inheriting the condition if one parent is affected, but the chances are better if the parents are older.

Medical Management
Wholly unsatisfactory. Hospitals may refuse to take such patients. Support and care at home is crucial but very difficult.

Social Management
Sex discrimination is very obvious; when the husband has the disease, his wife is expected to care for him, as an extension of her maternal role. When a wife is affected, the husband expects, and usually gets, help from social welfare agencies in order to cope.

Social Implications of the Disease
a   It is a repulsive condition, i.e. people are repelled by it.
b   Results in total physical and social dependence.
c   Leads to inability to relate to others, communication is lost and the patient and family are isolated.
d   Abnormal emotional atmosphere at home.
e   Intolerable burden on spouse, physically, emotionally and socially.
f   Stigma.

Genetic counselling
Desperately important, to reduce the numbers of people who will become affected. One of the most difficult conditions to face genetic counsellors.

Complications of the disorder
 1. Intercurrent infections.
 2. Unemployment.
 3. Divorce.
 4. **Suicide**.
 5. Arson.
 6. Murder.
 7. Sexual assaults/rape.
 8. Hypersexuality.
 9. Falls (fractures etc.).
10. Household damage
     — and innumerable others.

On a historical note: Known to have first occurred in an emigre family from the Boston area of Lincolnshire, who took it to the U.S.A. Well documented by the Huntingtons, a family of American doctors, through the early generations of the disorder. Now Huntington's Chorea is probably more common in the U.S.A. than in Britain.

Epilepsies

Definition
An **abnormal excessive** neuronal (electrical) discharge within the central nervous system. If it is sufficiently widespread, involves loss of consciousness and in certain forms convulsive seizures.

Idiopathic epilepsy
Of unknown cause. Very often of an hereditary basis. Could be of **petit-mal** type, **grand-mal** type or **Jacksonian**. It could also appear as a combination of all already mentioned.

Symptomatic or Secondary epilepsy
This type of epilepsy is a **symptom of an underlying disease**. Obviously more apparent when it appears for the first time in middle-age with no past history. Includes temporal-lobe epilepsy.

Underlying diseases
Can be divided into 2 categories:

a Intra-cranial   **b** Extra-cranial

a Intra-cranial

1. Space occupying lesions	e.g. cerebral tumours, abscesses.
2. Vascular lesions	e.g. acute and chronic cerebrovascular disease, cerebral thrombophlebitis, hypertensive encephalopathy.
3. Brain injury	e.g. at birth, resulting in atrophy and scarring of cerebral tissues.
4. Inflammatory disease	e.g. meningitis, encephalitis, G.P.I. meningo-vascular syphilis.
5. Degenerative disease	e.g. presenile dementia — Alzheimer's etc.

b Extra-cranial

1. Cerebral Anoxia	e.g. heart block, carbon-monoxide asphyxia.
2. Metabolic disturbances	e.g. uraemia, hypoglycaemia, alkalosis, hepatic failure.
3. Poisons	e.g. alcohol, lead, cardiazol, cocaine.
4. Undetermined causes	e.g. complication of teething in childhood. Increase in temperature.
5. Eclampsia	

Basic precipitating factors for all epilepsies
Emotional stress and conflict, fatigue, excitement, fever, hypoglycaemia, constipation, alcohol, increase in fluid intake, mental idleness, sensory stimuli, e.g. flickering lights.

The nurse's aim after the patient is admitted to hospital.
1. To assist the individual towards re-entry into as 'normal' a life as possible **a** in the community **b** within the hospital

2. To make thorough and continual medical observation possible so that the individual may receive the treatment most suitable for his needs.
3. To provide conditions under which convulsions and other symptoms are likely to diminish and mental deterioration may be prevented.
4. To protect the individual from harmful consequences of convulsions, e.g. punishment from actions over which they have no control (when in epileptic fugue or furor).

Nursing care
Prevention
1. Physical: To maintain the patient's general health at the highest level possible, e.g. avoid internal irritation such as constipation, infections. Avoid hypoglycaemia and alkalosis — regulate the diet, e.g. if the patient is known to have convulsions during the night, allow them to have a snack before going to bed. Decrease fluid intake. Ensure that the patient takes **regular medication**.

2. Psychological: Relieve mental stress and conflict. Reduce anxiety. Tact, encouragement, support.

Observation: Side effects of drugs used.

Phenobarbitone	Drowsiness.
Mysoline	Drowsiness, vertigo, ataxia, diplopa, skin rashes, megaloblastic anaemia.
Phenytoin	Gastric upset, dermatitis, hypertrophy and hypertension of the gums. Nystagmus and ataxia, megaloblastic anaemia, leucopenia, agranulocytosis, depression, intellectual deterioration, peripheral neuropathy.
Carbamazepine	Drowsiness, skin reactions, dry mouth, etc.

Accurate, detailed report of convulsions
1. Time.
2. External circumstances at the time.
3. Mental condition before convulsion.
4. Whether or not onlookers present.
5. Onset.

6. Any complaints by patient.
7. State of consciousness.
8. Muscular movements.
9. Cyanosis.
10. Incontinence.
11. Injury to body.
12. Mental and physical condition after convulsion.
13. Unusual behaviour.

Management of convulsions (seizures)

Convulsions (seizures) may be **localized** e.g. petit-mal, Jacksonian, or **generalized** (grand-mal). Very little can be done in the nurse's role with regard to petit-mal or Jacksonian convulsions except to observe and report accurately.

Grand-Mal convulsion

1. **Aura** Usually occurs in symptomatic epilepsy. This phase may or may not occur. It can take many forms: tension, irritability, hallucinations, 'queer' sensations — abdominal, smell etc. Many individuals suffering from epilepsy who experience this phase are to make themselves 'comfortable' before the following stages.
2. **Tonic phase** 'Epileptic cry', due to contraction of the respiratory muscles. Loss of consciousness — rigidity depends on which are the strongest muscles. The back may be arched, arms flexed, fists clenched with the thumbs in the palms. Legs are stiff, with the feet turned inward. Respiration stops, the patient becomes cyanosed. The face becomes contorted with eyes open, appearing to be to one side or upwards. The pupils are dilated, (no reaction to light). The phase lasts 5 to 40 seconds.
3. **Clonic phase** Rigidity disappears gradually, muscles relax, jerky movements of face, trunk, arms and legs. Tongue may be bitten, froth at the mouth. Patient appears flushed with profuse perspiration. There is possible incontinence. The phase lasts 40 to 60 seconds.
4. **Flaccid coma** (recovery stage) Jerking gradually stops, the muscles are completely relaxed (flaccid), breathing is deep and noisy, there may be occasional vomiting. Headache, confusion, drowsiness — comatosed state.

Complications

Injuries may occur as listed below.

a Tongue biting (tonic-clonic phase).
b Falling — depends what the individual is doing and where he happens to be, e.g. fire, hard objects etc.

c Dislocations — mainly of shoulders and jaws.
d Status epilepticus — one convulsion following another, resulting in fatigue, exhaustion, cardiac failure, pneumonia etc.

Important points to be carried out
a Restrain only if there is possibility of injury.
b Maintain clear airway (turn head to one side).
c Prevent biting of tongue — mouth gag or rolled up cloth placed at angle of mouth.
d Should another convulsion occur, inform Medical Officer.

Temporal Lobe Epilepsy

The symptoms vary depending on the area affected. One or more of the following may be affected:

1. Epigastric sensation: unpleasant sensation in pit of stomach, chest and throat.
2. Changes of perception: objects appear smaller (micropsia) or larger (macropsia), dimmer or brighter. Sounds seem louder or more distant.
3. Hallucinations: olfactory, gustatory, visual or auditory.
4. Changes in the quality of familiarity: disturbance of memory.
5. Changes of thought: time rushing by or standing still. Repetition of words, music etc.
6. Dreamy states: feelings of unreality, depersonalisation.
7. Primary automatism: may go through the same set of actions, e.g. dressing etc.
8. Affective disorders: disorders of mood, e.g. pleasure, anxiety, terror, depression, paranoia, aggression etc.

Effects of Epilepsy

1. Epileptic personality
Changes of personality — slowness, rigidity in thinking and reaction, self-centred, hypochondriacal.
Fixed attitudes and opinions.
Deterioration — dementia.
Irritable, quarrelsome, aggressive.

2. Schizophrenia-like psychoses

Pre-Senile Dementias

Pre-Senile Dementia affects the intellectual function and emotional response in adults of the age group 40 to 65 years. The dementia is due to organic cerebral change.

1. Alzheimer's Disease

This condition usually occurs in the 5th decade. The onset of the disease is gradual, but in the later stages there is a severe degree of dementia. Plaques are laid down and the brain atrophies.

2. Pick's Disease

Atrophy of the brain occurs which is more localised in the frontal and temporal regions. The neurones swell and balloon out. The disease progresses slowly with death occurring after 5 to 10 years. Only a post-mortem on a patient can prove whether he was suffering from Alzheimer's or Pick's Disease.

3. Huntington's Chorea

This is an hereditary disease which usually manifests itself in the 3rd to 4th decade. It begins with choreiform movements due to degeneration of the Basal Ganglia. A progressive dementia follows. Death occurs within 10 to 20 years of onset. Because this disease does not manifest itself until the 3rd or 4th decade, the patient may have already passed the disease to her or his children.

See also separate section on this disorder.

4. Jacob-Creutzfeldt Disease

This illness starts with vague physical discomforts. After a few weeks, the dementing process begins and runs a rapid course. Death usually occurs within 3 to 9 months of onset.

Treatment
The treatment of pre-senile dementia is symptomatic.

Arteriopathic disease

Types of Arteriosclerosis

1. *Aterosclerosis:* affects large and small vessels — aorta, coronaries, small vessels at the base of the brain in particular. The internal coat is affected — atheromatous plaques leading to thrombosis.
2. *Arterio-capillary sclerosis:* small vessels of kidney and spleen, liver, pancreas and muscles affected, but those of heart and lungs escape.
3. *Monckeberg's sclerosis:* not a cause of increased blood pressure. Medial coat affected — calcified — pipe stem arteries. Affects mainly the arteries of the legs in old people. Causes intermittent claudication and gangrene of toes.

Arteriosclerosis is not a prerequisite for high blood pressure cf. Cushing's Syndrome, tumours of adrenals (phaeochromocytomata) and renal insufficiency.

Essential Hypertension, i.e. increased blood pressure not due to arteriosclerosis but often associated with it. It is, however, causative of arteriosclerosis. In most cases there is a family history of essential hypertension.

Malignant Hypertension. Increased B.P. in younger people causes papilloedema — kidney failure — death rapid.

Simple Hypertension. Increased B.P. in older subjects, kidney symptoms — papilloedema.

Relationship between Hypertension and Arteriosclerosis

1. *Essential*   Benign 90%
              Malignant 10%
2. *Secondary*: to Cushing's Disease, adrenal tumours, polycystic kidney etc.

Hypertension causes reactive thickening of arterial wall. Obesity, etc. contributes. Little connection between retinal and peripheral sclerosis and cerebral vascular sclerosis.

Effects of arteriosclerosis on the brain

1. Softening and haemorrhage.
2. Granular atrophy of cortex.

Clinical features of Cerebral Arteriopathic Dementia

Usually begins in the sixties, but occasionally as early as the forties. In about half the cases it is preceded by cerebrovascular accident. Usually there is an acute delirious episode, failing memory, emotional, inclination to wander at night. Headaches, giddiness, palpitations, momentary black-outs. Memory loss for recent events often the first symptom — diaries kept — Korsakow's Syndrome. Difficulty in concentration, inefficient, narrowing of outlook. Judgement and basic personality well preserved, good insight, causes despondency and depression with pessimism. Emotional incontinence (cf. pseudo Bulbar palsy). Slower intellectual impairment than in senile dementia, but more distinctive feature is the *marked fluctuation in the course of the illness.* Determined suicide attempts are likely in delirious episodes with depressive colouring, but a few hours afterwards, the patient is often euphoric and oblivious.

Somatic symptoms

Headache, giddiness, tinnitus, general malaise, praecordial discomfort.

Neurological

Aphasias, hemiparesis (transient or permanent), visual field defects. Epileptic fits, 15-20%.

Minor C.N.S. abnormalities — sluggish pupils, abnormal reflexes.

The fluctuating course of the disease is maintained to a late stage.

Death due to
(Cerebro vascular accident
(Cardiac failure
(Pneumonia

Prognosis
70% of patients are dead in two years.

Treatment
1. 2–3 weeks complete rest
2. Slimming, reduced salt intake, vitamins
3. Adequate sleep
4. Reassurance
5. Restrict responsibilities
6. Hypotensive drugs
7. E.C.T. may be necessary if a depressive, agitated picture develops.
8. Early discharge home — if at all possible.

Prognosis
30% recover
35% die
35% hospital in-patients

Delirious States
Acute attacks of clouded consciousness common in old age. May occur as exacerbation of organic process, e.g. arteriosclerosis, or early senile dementia; also may announce:

1. cerebral neoplasm
2. G.P.I.
3. cardiac failure
4. chronic subdural haematoma
5. after operation, especially cataract and prostatectomy
6. respiratory infections

Prognosis
40% die
55% recover
Few remain in hospital

Psychological changes in old age

Introductory points

1. Being 'psychologically old' means thinking and feeling and behaving in a particular way. It does not mean that one has reached any particular age.
2. The 'normal' changes in the thinking of 'old' people are those which are shown by most people. They are not those which 'ought' to happen, or which we would like to happen, simply those, which, in fact, do happen.
3. The 'abnormal' changes are those which do not happen to most of us, and which may, therefore, be regarded as evidence of 'illness' or 'disease'.
4. The difference between the 'normal' and the 'abnormal' is often (but not always) a matter of degree; in many cases it is difficult to draw a clear outline between the two.
5. In addition to the psychological, there are physical, sociological and spiritual aspects of 'old age'.

Normal old age

Fundamentally the psychological changes may be summed up in a phrase 'a progressive lessening of efficiency in all spheres of mental activity; accompanied by compensatory behaviour patterns aimed at minimising the effects of the inefficiency'.

The inabilities
a *Intellectual* leading to an inability to register new events:
   (i) difficulty in comprehension and acceptance of new ideas
   (ii) memory disturbance — recent memory lost, distant memory retained
   (iii) narrowing of interest — self-centredness
b *Emotional* leading to an inability to feel deeply or consistently:
   (i) rapid changes from one emotion to another
   (ii) absence of emotional 'infectiousness'
c *Behaviour* leading to an inability to inhibit:
   (i) disregard of conventional behaviour, e.g. table manners
   (ii) lessened control over sphincters
   (iii) irritability and fault finding

The Compensations

Routine way of life	— to minimise occurrence of new events.
Reliance of reminiscence	— to perpetuate occurrence of old events.
Hoarding	
Projection of one's shortcomings onto others	— to prevent the realisation of the
Confabulation	inefficiencies.

Abnormal old age
1. **Senile Dementia** — the ultimate end result
   Total disorientation
   Total dependence   back to the starting point
   Total depersonalisation
2. **Arteriopathic Dementia**
   Dementia and neurological evidence of arteriopathic brain disease, occurring in 'younger' people with better preserved personalities and running a fluctuating course.
3. **Senile delirium**
   Acute confusion with hallucinosis — a toxic-infective phenomena, associated with malnutrition and avitaminosis.
4. **'Senile' Melancholia**
   Two types
   a Angeric (retarded) manic-depressive depression
   b Agitated (involutional) melancholia

Two special points
a) Physical dysfunction and pain may commonly be the presenting symptom.
b) The preoccupation with morbid thoughts may produce the picture of pseudo-dementia.
5. **Late Paraphrenia**
   Delusional psychosis with preservation of the personality often associated with sensory deprivation.

Practice Questions

1. What are the main features of dementia?
2. Name three causes of dementia.
3. What is the incidence of puerperal psychosis?
4. What is 'Folie a deux'?
5. What is the difference between Huntington's Chorea and Sydenham's Chorea?
6. How common is Huntington's Chorea?
7. Name four complications of Huntington's Chorea.
8. What is the meaning of the word 'idiopathic'?
9. What are the four stages which occur in a classical epileptic fit?
10. What are the dangers to the patient resulting from status epilepticus?
11. What is micropsia?
12. Name two forms of pre-senile dementia.
13. What is the prognosis for patients suffering from Jacob-Creutzfeldt disease?
14. What is the usual cause of death in a case of malignant hypertension?
15. What is meant by emotional lability?
16. To what does the term 'involutional' refer?

17. What is paraphrenia?
18. The onset of puerperal psychosis is usually:
    a rather sudden
    b insidious
    c only pre-natally
    d only post-natally
19. What percentage of patients suffering from puerperal psychosis have had a previous history of mental disorder?
    a 10%
    b 20%
    c 30%
    d more than 50%
20. Flexibilitas cerea occurs most commonly in which type of schizophrenia?
    a simple
    b paranoid
    c hebephrenic
    d catatonic
21. Where one parent suffers from Hungtington's Chorea, the chances of a child suffering the same condition are:
    a even
    b 1 in 4
    c 1 in 8
    d 1 in 16.
22. Huntington's Chorea usually manifests itself:
    a at birth
    b during childhood
    c in the 3rd or 4th decade
    d in old age.
23. In Monckeberg's Sclerosis the part of the artery affected is:
    a tunica adventitia
    b tunica intima
    c tunica media
    d all of these.
24. The memory defect which classically occurs in old age is:
    a transient
    b anterograde
    c retrograde
    d intermittent.
25. In senile dementia, the personality is usually:
    a well preserved
    b complete, though changed
    c poorly preserved
    d totally lost.

Answers on page 46.

Answers

 1. All mental processes are involved, especially cognition, affect and behaviour. The clinical picture varies from patient to patient.
 2. Three causes may be taken from the following: systemic infections, inflammatory conditions of the Central Nervous System, head injury, epilepsy, space-occupying lesions, drugs including alcohol, cerebral anoxia, uraemia, liver failure.
 3. 1 in 50.
 4. Folie à deux is a 'communicated insanity' resulting from a sympathetic reaction to a disorder suffered by another person. Usually the secondary sufferer has strong emotional ties with the 'real' patient.
 5. Huntington's Chorea is a serious genetic disorder with death occurring 15 to 20 years after the onset. Sydenham's Chorea is a childhood condition, once called St. Vitus' Dance, and is associated with rheumatism.
 6. Probably greater than 1 in 4000.
 7. Suicide, intercurrent infections, falls and fractures, criminal behaviour.
 8. Idiopathic simply means of 'unknown cause'.
 9. 1. Aura. 2. Tonic stage. 3. Clonic stage. 4. Recovery stage.
10. Exhaustion and death.
11. Literally, seeing small things; a subjective perception where objects appear smaller than normal, common in temporal lobe epilepsy.
12. Pick's Disease. Alzheimer's Disease. Huntington's Chorea. Jacob-Creutzfeldt disease.
13. Very poor indeed. The usual course of the disease is from onset to death within twelve months.
14. Renal failure.
15. Rapid changes of emotional state.
16. Involutional, as in involutional melancholia, refers to the menopause.
17. Paraphrenia is usually regarded as late-onset schizophrenia, with a well preserved personality and a comparatively good prognosis.
18. Rather sudden
20. Catatonic
21. Even
22. In the 3rd or 4th decade.
23. Tunica media
24. Anterograde
25. Totally lost

5 PSYCHONEUROSIS

The aim of this chapter is to acquaint the nurse with the nature of psychoneurosis and how it affects the individual. Included here is a section on personality disorders, which, strictly, are not neuroses, but they resemble neurotic conditions more closely than psychotic disorders.

The objectives of this chapter are:
a To describe anxiety, reactive depression, phobia, hysteria and obsessional neurosis.
b To present the features, types and treatment of the commoner forms of personality disorder.

Psychoneurosis

For the general nurse, psychoneurosis may be very difficult to understand and have sympathy for, since no active disease process is at work. Nonetheless, some forms of neurosis can be highly incapacitating and cause the patient immense stress. Neurosis arises due to a defect of personality which may be traceable to the patient's upbringing, or may be of completely unknown and of untraceable origin.

To some extent we are all neurotic. Elements within our personalities cause us to over-react to events, or occasion stress or un-toward behaviour in certain circumstances. These we can pass off as manifestations of our individuality, or as eccentricities, and rarely do they cause any lasting or serious problem. Generally they do not call for treatment, nor do they interfere with out pursuit of happiness or prevent us from doing our jobs. When, however, these personality 'quirks' develop to a pathological degree causing us misery, fear, anguish and affecting our behaviour to an intolerable level, a state very akin to a true illness exists.

The incidence of neurosis is high; how high, we do not know, but G.P.s see more neurotic patients in their surgeries than any other group of medical disorders. Anxiety states and neurotic depression are common, hysteria and obsessional states less so.

Anxiety states
Anxiety is felt by everyone, usually in a mild form, in threatening circumstances. To an extent it is beneficial, anxiety being the 'main-

spring of action'. In anxiety neurosis, however, the anxiety is either excessive or inappropriate to the circumstances. The physical manifestations of anxiety are those of an excess of adrenaline. The autonomic nervous system is hyperactive, causing palpitations, gastric upsets, sweating, trembling, headache, diarrhoea and insomnia.

The patient feels tense, worried, apprehensive and unable to concentrate; primarily the feeling is of fear, though he does not know, in some cases, of what it is he is frightened, the so-called 'free-floating anxiety' state. The condition may be persistent and chronic, or may occur as sporadic attacks of acute anxiety (panic attack) which may last for minutes or hours. For the previously stable person, who experiences a panic attack on occasions, the outlook is good, but for the 'anxious personality', who experiences the longer-lasting free-floating anxiety, the prognosis is less satisfactory. Commonly, such patients develop one or more of a host of psychosomatic disorders, and are then seen more commonly in general hospitals than in psychiatric hospitals. It is usually the element of depression, which often accompanies anxiety, which may lead to the admission of a patient to a psychiatric hospital.

E.C.T. is not the treatment of choice as the depressive component of the disorder is of the neurotic rather than psychotic variety. Rather, antidepressives, anxietiolytics and minor tranquillisers may be prescribed. These, together with supportive psychotherapy, are the mainstay of treatment.

Phobia States (See also under Child/Adolescent psychiatry)
These are forms of anxiety state, but the fear the patient experiences is focussed and well-known to the patient. The fear is out of all proportion and appears quite unreasonable to a non-afflicted observer. No voluntary control of this fear is possible, and it leads to the patient avoiding the feared object or situation at all costs.

Sometimes the object of fear is not so unreasonable, e.g. cancer, venereal disease, but the degree and severity of the fear is out of proportion. In other cases, the fear is of objects which are normally considered neutral and entirely harmless, e.g. birds, leaves. Many perfectly normal people have a distaste for certain things, not amounting to a phobia, e.g. heights, slugs, snakes and spiders; such distaste is not however incapacitating, nor do we find our lives dominated by the need to avoid them.

The range of phobias is truly astounding, from the commonest, agoraphobia, to stranger objects of fear such as trees, flowers, sleep, cessation of breathing, children, foreigners, women, food, work, sunlight, even everything (panphobia).

The 'Housebound Housewife' (Agoraphobia)

The commonest phobia; 75% of those affected are women. It may well constitute the most common neurosis in women. The patient's condition usually begins in early adult life, shortly after marriage, and manifests itself as a fear of leaving the house, of open streets, of travelling, public places and meeting other people.

The patient experiences dizziness, panic attacks, depression and nausea in these circumstances. The condition tends to run a chronic course and persists for many years. The patient's husband and children become involved at an early stage, and the patient soon learns that there is a certain secondary gain in her condition.

In hospital, using conditioning, or behaviour modification techniques, the patient may do well, but commonly, on return home, reverts to her original state. Merely treating the phobia is of little lasting avail; the underlying cause is her neurotic personality and this requires longer-term support and treatment.

The condition should be differentiated from **Social Phobia**, again common, and women are the main sufferers. Shy, sensitive ladies find themselves paralysingly afraid of some social situations, e.g. eating/drinking in public, speaking in public, attending parties or using public toilets. The prognosis is better than for true agoraphobics.

Hysteria

The name Hysteria is of Greek origin and originally implied a condition of the womb (uterus); hysterectomy has the same origin. Since the condition was thought to be exclusive to women, it was reasoned to be a disorder of some female organ. Men, however, **do** suffer from hysteria, though predominantly it is still considered to be a female disorder.

The term 'Hysteria' is used in several different ways.

a When a person is out of control and reacting in irrational ways we say they are hysterical.

b Certain people have hysterical personalities.

c Loss of physiological functions without organic disease is called 'Conversion Hysteria'. It is the patient's method of dealing with stress, although she is unaware of the reason and mechanism.

d When an organic condition is present, she, the patient, may exaggerate the condition and exploit it for her own ends. We call this 'Hysterical Overlay'.

Hysterical Personality

Some people indulge in behaviour which is histrionic. They are usually emotionally immature; like children, they are unable to control their emotions, and they are very self-centred (egocentricity) and demanding of attention. They often have a remarkable talent for self-deception. This person **feels** more than other people do; her mood states swing wildly from excess to excess. Immediately aroused enthusiasms are just as quickly lost as her attention swings to some seemingly more profitable area of self-display. She dresses ostentatiously and makes her moods and her physical presence patently obvious to all around her. She is typified as the gushing hostess surrounded by her admirers, over-loud, gesturing and addressing everyone around her as 'darling'. Whilst she may appear to be happy with her histrionics, she is wholly at the mercy of her vacillating moods. In the theatrical profession she may be an asset; elsewhere she is just tiresome.

Conversion Hysteria

Physical dysfunction in the absence of organic damage may occur as a result of overwhelming stress in a hitherto normal person, but is more likely to occur in those of a hysterical personality.

In **malingering** the person simulates a disorder in order to gain from it, and he knows exactly what he is doing thereby. In Conversion Hysteria, the simulation is similar, but the patient may genuinely be unaware of the mechanism. Were the patient to attend her G.P. with complaints of stress, inability to cope, or need for human attention, she would expect, and get, little sympathy. Rather, she presents with a **physical** dysfunction. Both the doctor and those around her well understand physical abnormalities; sympathy and attention are given accordingly.

The range of dysfunctions she may exhibit is very large, and includes paralysis of limbs, anaesthesia of the 'glove and stocking' variety, blindness, aphonia, total amnesia and pseudo-dementia. The condition often appears strange, since it accords with what the patient thinks the disease is like. Hence hysterical fits are wild thrashings about while gurgling and screaming, unlike the classical pattern of the epileptic fit. Our Victorian great grandmothers had attacks of 'the vapours', wherein they collapsed slowly and gracefully to the carpet to become unconscious until they received the attention they deemed appropriate. More often they collapsed on a handy bed or sofa, these being softer than carpets.

The attention the hysteric gains from her dysfunctions more than makes up for the inconvenience, and there is a phenomenon known as 'la belle indifference' where the person talks lightly of her condition, almost disregarding it.

These often demanding patients may evoke hostility in those who have to deal with them. Certainly it is difficult to maintain sympathy whilst denying them the attention they seek in order not to reinforce their belief that they are indeed physically ill.

Obsessional neurosis

We are all familiar with the tune we cannot get out of our minds. This is a minor obsession, and is a common occurrence in children and young people. Similarly, we remember going to school perhaps and en route performing rather pointless acts such as touching every tree in the avenue or avoiding treading upon the cracks in the pavement. These motor acts are called **Compulsions**, since we felt strangely compelled to perform them. In their minor states, these obsessions and compulsions are no more than a temporary nuisance and we tend to grow out of them. For an unhappy few, however, they increase to become a major neurosis, highly distressing to the individual, who knows only too well that they are pointless. In extreme cases they come to dominate his life, and suicide is a grave risk. This is the condition Sigmund Freud called **Zwangneurose**, in Britain it is called **Obsessional Neurosis** and in the U.S.A. it is called **Compulsive Neurosis**. Often we combine both terms to call it **Obsessional-compulsive Neurosis**, though this is something of a tautology.

Psychopathology

Normally as we progress from childhood to adulthood we adapt to the demands that society makes and suppress our own wants and wishes to a balanced and acceptable extent. For some, however, society's demands are ruthlessly instilled into the growing child by perhaps over-zealous parents, and the child's wish to do what is right. In yet other children there will be a 'Reaction Formation' and the child will reject or ignore society's demands and go his own defiant way.

Hence the development of certain characteristics in these groups of children:

a Orderliness, parsimony, obedience, tidiness, meticulosity and punctuality — all result from excessive obedience to parents' (society's) demands.
b Obstinacy, defiance, challenging, radicalism — all result from rejection of parents' demands.

The former type of child develops an obsessional personality; not ill and not handicapped by his excessive conformity, but his life is characterised by being fastidious, orderly, tidy, fussy, punctual, rigid, pedantic and just-so. Commonly, too, he will be irritable, bad-tempered and somewhat aggressive. Many of these characteristics can be channelled into socially acceptable outlets, particularly if his work is concerned with precision, e.g. watchmaking, precision engineering or book-keeping.

For the unfortunate few of these 'obsessive personalities', these characteristics develop to a pathological degree with superstitions, fears, religiosity, ceremonies, observances and meticulous rituals, progressing to phobias of dirt, disease and animals etc. Obsessional ideas and images continually plague his mind and these take the form of ruminations on religious, metaphysical, philosophical and pseudo-scientific themes. These are particularly distressing if they are nonsensical:

> 'Ah, Man; wherefore does he why? And whither does he wither?'
> 'Punch, brothers, punch with care,
> Punch in the presence of the passenjair'

Compulsions follow obsessions. Ritual handwashing follows a 'dirt' obsession, endlessly repeated. Obsessions of doubt are common (folie le doute). 'Did I close the door?', followed by endless returning to check — although he knows he did. Exactitude in all acts is aimed at, but never attained. Anxiety and tension are ever present. The range and persistence of symptoms can be mild to totally incapacitating.

The tendency to resist these obsessions and compulsions is virtually diagnostic, but the resistance is unsuccessful. He is certainly not helped by the propensity of others to tell him to desist, 'think of something else' or 'pull himself together'.

Age group
15–25 years at onset is a common finding.

Differential diagnosis
Normal child rituals.
Fatigue, physical ill-health.
Depression.
Schizophrenia.
Phobia/Anxiety states.

Complications
Work, family and social disorganisation.
Sleeplessness, fatigue, exhaustion and death.
Suicide.

Treatment
Phenothiazines.
Intensive psychotherapy.
Apotreptic (aversion) therapy.
Behaviour modification.
Abreaction is contra-indicated.

In nursing these patients, ritual prevention is commonly tried, but is rarely effective, and may well cause the patient to be further distressed. The converse, i.e. ordering the patient to perform the rituals, may well be more effective, since although he cannot resist his own inner compulsion to perform the rituals, he may well be able to resist your orders. In any case, after half a life-time of being told by others to desist, it is refreshing (and therapeutic) to be allowed and encouraged to abandon resistance.

The endless patience and genuine sympathy of the nursing staff is required in caring for this acutely distressed and mentally tortured patient. The condition may well become intolerable to the patient, and suicide is a serious and ever-present risk. In such cases, psychosurgery, in the form of pre-frontal leucotomy, may be the last and only hope of releasing the patient from what is, arguably, the most unpleasant and distressing mental illness of all.

Personality Disorders

This refers to a group of fairly well defined anomalies or deviations of personality which are not the result of a psychosis or of any other illness. These traits have been present since an early age and are frequently attributed to unhealthy upbringing. This group of disorders is categorized according to which personality traits are most prominent.

1. **Paranoid**
   Here there is an excessive tendency to self-reference and suspiciousness. Two types:
   a Sensitive and vulnerable people who react excessively to the average daily experiences of life with a sense of subjection and humiliation and who tend to blame others for their experiences.
   b More aggressive people who are excessively sensitive of what they conceive to be their rights. They are vulnerable to any violation of these rights and are tenacious in their defence.

2. **Affective (Cyclothymic)**
   Personalities who have persistent anomalies of mood. They vary from the depressed to the hypermanic. These symptoms frequently fluctuate in the same individual.

3. Schizoid
Here there is aloofness, shyness and reserve. They are introspective people, making few social contacts.

4. Anankastic (Obsessive-Compulsive or Obsessional Personality)
These are cautious, conforming, conscientious people. They are extremely meticulous and are perfectionists. If they fall from these high standards, they frequently have feelings of guilt.

5. Hysterical
These are shallow labile, over-dependent people, craving love and attention. They are showy demonstrative people, tending to over-dramatize things. Their relationship with other people is usually unreliable. Under stress, they develop hysterical symptoms.

6. Asthenic (Inadequate personality)
These people lack mental vigour and stamina. They find great difficulty in dealing with the normal ups and downs of life. Under these stresses, they frequently develop symptoms of anxiety and depression and make frequent suicide attempts.

7. Antisocial
People who offend against society, who show lack of sympathetic feelings, and their behaviour is not modified by experience or punishment. They are cold, callous people, prone to aggressive and irresponsible conduct.

Psychopathy
No universal definitions. Various definitions have four features:

1. Description of behaviour:	Antisocial, impulsive, irresponsible, aggressive and criminal.
2. Personality characteristics:	Egocentricity, lack of sincerity, lack of feeling, unaware of effect on others and lack of guilt.
3. Time factor:	from early life — recurrent episodic or persistent.
4. Excluding cause:	no mental defect, no mental illness (psychosis or neurosis) or brain damage.

Mental Health Act 1959 defines it as a Persistent Disorder of Personality (whether or not accompanied by subnormality of intelligence) which results in abnormally aggressive or seriously irresponsible conduct on the part of the patient and requires or is susceptible to medical treatment.

A convenient definition is a person who has shown from an early age an abnormality of character marked by episodes of anti-social behaviour and tendencies to act on impulse to satisfy the need of the moment, without due regard to the consequences of such action.

Views on its Aetiology
1. Organic defect of moral sense — moral insanity.
2. Hereditary basis. Great conflict here of genetic versus environmental.
3. Sociological approach. Patient might have been brought up in a psychopathic subculture.
4. Reparative behaviour — compensating for feelings of inadequacy and inferiority.
5. Psychodynamic approach.
   Weak ego verses strong id.
   Defective upbringing — poor behavioural standards provided by parents.
   Arrested development — child-like state persisting.
6. Organic brain disease.
   Deviant behaviour with minimal brain damage. Birth trauma.
   Sometimes Temporal Lobe Epilepsy may produce psychopathic behaviour.
   E.E.G. may be abnormal.

Treatment
1. Physical — very limited.
2. Individual psychotherapy — unrewarding.
3. Group therapy — may be useful.
4. Therapeutic Community — Henderson Hospital.
   Four main social factors are at work in the Therapeutic Community:
   a Communalism in sharing of tasks, responsibilities and rewards.
   b Democratic decision making.
   c Permissiveness to act in accord with one's feelings without accustomed social inhibitions.
   d Confrontation of the subject with what he has done by the group in the 'here and now'.

The very difficult are in special Prison Hospitals: Broadmoor, Rampton, Moss Side and Park Lane Hospitals.

Natural History and Prognosis
? Treatable
? Burns out in time. Picture less overt, but are destructive in the family.
Death by violence or suicide is common.

Practice Questions

1. Give three physical manifestations of anxiety.
2. What is the difference between free-floating anxiety and phobia?
3. Name at least ten objects of fear for phobic patients.
4. What is thought to be the commonest form of neurosis in women?
5. What is conversion hysteria?
6. Sigmund Freud referred to obsessional neurosis as . . .?
7. Name three occupations which are more likely to be suited to persons suffering from obsessional neurosis.
8. What is the most serious complication of obsessional neurosis?
9. What are the general features of psychopathy?
10. Name two of the four Special Hospitals in England.

Answers on page 58.

Answers

1. Diarrhoea, gastric upsets, palpitations, dry mouth, tremor, gooseflesh, hypertension.
2. In free-floating anxiety, the patient is unaware of a reason for his anxiety, whereas in phobic states, the patient is able to pinpoint a definite object of fear.
3. The list is virtually endless, but could contain: open spaces, spiders, snakes, slugs, insects, dogs, cats, birds, dirt, leaves, infection, cancer, children, men, women, sex, sleep, falling, rain, sunshine, thunder, colours, darkness, dreams, poison, aeroplanes, noise, quietness. Agoraphobia is by far the most common.
4. Agoraphobia.
5. Conversion hysteria is a form of neurosis where the patient's psychological state is converted into physical dysfunctions.
6. Zwangneurose.
7. Among occupations suited to persons with obsessional neurosis are watchmaking, precision engineering, book-keeping, precision assembly work, technical illustration.
8. Suicide.
9. General features of psychopathy are antisocial behaviour, egocentricity, irresponsibility, lack of guilt, inability to benefit from experience, e.g. from punishment.
10. Moss Side, Park Lane, Broadmoor, Rampton.

6   CHILD AND ADOLESCENT PSYCHIATRY

Child and adolescent psychiatry is mainly concerned with behaviour disorders, difficulties in social adaptation and forms of neurotic and psychotic reactions. It is vital that the child and adolescent is recognised as a changing personality influenced by psychological factors, and in need of affection, discipline, security and understanding by his parents. Problems very often arise from a combination of factors, i.e. emotional and situational ones; also, in some cases, from intellectual and constitutional causes. The patient is usually seen at Child Guidance/Assessment Clinics or Adolescent Units usually annexed to a psychiatric hospital. Within a general hospital, the nurse is most likely to encounter child and adolescent problems in a Casualty Department or a Paediatric Ward.

The objectives of this section are:

a   To outline the possible causes of child/adolescent crises.
b   To describe briefly some of the common psychiatric/psychosocial problems seen in children and adolescents.
c   To outline the nursing and psychiatric management of patients suffering from child and adolescent crises.

Causes of Child/Adolescent Crises

1. Genetic factors, i.e. Infantile Autism, Schizophreniform disorders resembling adult Schizophrenia.
2. Parent/child relationships, i.e. parental instability, maternal deprivation, maternal oversolicitude.
3. Parental discord/disharmony, i.e. marital problems may have repercussions on the child's development.
4. Sibling-rivalry. It has been suggested that Anorexia Nervosa may result from rivalry between siblings — but see also under Schizophrenia.
5. One-parent family.
6. The only child — over-protection by parents may be unhealthy for the child. Over-dependence on parents may be a handicap for later development.
7. Parents with psychiatric disorders — children and adolescents may suffer psychosocial problems as a result of an abnormal environment.

8. Socialisation process — the lack of which may result in shyness and difficulty to relate at a later stage of development.
9. Trauma, i.e. brain-injured child.
10. Drug abuse, especially in the adolescent, experimenting with glue sniffing and drugs of addiction.

Childhood/Adolescent Crises

1. Psychotic Disorders

Infantile autism
Usually occurs before three years of age — the child manifests deficits in language development, problems of socialisation, bizarre responses to his environment, hyperkinesis, stereotyped movements, fears and self-destructive and self-punitive behaviour. There is an absence of delusions and hallucinations.

Schizophrenic syndromes
Rarely occur before the age of seven, bear some resemblance to adult Schizophrenia, but difficult to diagnose.

2. Neurotic Disorders
Although neurotic disorders among children and adolescents are not seen in psychiatric hospitals, it is true to say that Anxiety states, Phobias, Depression (Reactive), Obsessional-Compulsive Neuroses and Hysteria can be seen in some forms. However, these manifestations can be difficult to diagnose at the initial onset.

Habit disturbances
These include repetitive activities such as temper tantrums, tics, nail-biting, thumb-sucking, masturbation, enuresis, head-rolling and stammering. These conditions are primarily auto-erotic and probably suggest a form of regression.

Enuresis: a common condition encountered by the child/adolescent psychiatrist. At the age of between 2 and 3 most children would have ceased to wet themselves. Enuresis occurs twice as frequently in boys as in girls. By far the most common form of enuresis is the nocturnal type, but it is possible to develop the diurnal type, together with nocturnal enuresis. In the majority of cases, no evidence of organic disorders of the nervous system or genito-urinary system is seen. Enuresis can arise from inadequate training, maternal over-protectiveness and attention-seeking, or as a result of a new-born child in the family.

Treatment is usually effected by conditioning and use of Anti-Depressants, e.g. Imipramine, 25 to 50 mg at night for older children. Most cases do recover before adult life.

School Phobia (School refusal)
Common between the ages of 5 and 12 years. In most instances, it is not related to school, but due to separation from mother — a form of separation anxiety. Mothers are often over-protective and over-anxious. The child, usually a boy, manifests symptoms of abdominal pain, nausea and vomiting, which result in refusal to attend school. The most effective forms of treatment are the following.
a   Ignoring the child's physical complaints.
b   Individual and family psychotherapy.
c   Assessing school problems, if any.
d   Forced school attendance.

Success Depression
Really a form of reactive depression, this is common among adolescents between the ages 15 and 18. It is closely related to scholastic achievement, in which the adolescent is constantly being pressurised by his parents to attain certain unusually high levels of achievement. Adolescents whose academic potentials cannot be stretched to beyond their normal limit usually become depressed and in some cases suicidal.

Treatment is geared to improving understanding between the parents and the adolescent, together with assistance from teachers. Anti-Depressant drugs may be of value in the acute stage.

3. Conduct Disorders
These relate to behavioural aberrations seen in both children and adolescents, and present a growing concern to parents. It is usually first noticeable in the home or school surroundings by parents and teachers. The behaviour manifested by the child or adolescent is against the normative standard approved by society, and therefore lends itself to legal implications.

Juvenile delinquency is very common among cliques or groups of children. It seems to be an ego-boosting exercise in terms of belonging to a particular group. It takes various forms, e.g. stealing, arson, general destructiveness etc. Most of these activities take place in urban areas, but recently have spread to rural regions as well. It is difficult to isolate one particular cause of delinquency; it is usually a combination of disturbed family background and subcultural influences, especially in school and large families.

4. Anorexia Nervosa

A common and increasing problem of adolescent girls, but very uncommon in the male population — 1 in 150 males may suffer from this condition as compared with a staggering 1 in 20 girls during the adolescent period. Common features are:

a Anorexia: literally means loss of appetite, but such patients *are* hungry, though suppressing their hunger.

b Loss of weight and energy.

c Self-induced vomiting.

d Amenorrhoea.

e Constipation.

Intensive treatment is vital in the early stages. Very often, treatment is resisted by the patient, and if this happens, the prognosis is poor and death may ensue. Close observation, use of phenothiazines, individual and family psychotherapy and behaviour modification are strategies used in the management of anorexics.

Further notes on Anorexia Nervosa are given in the chapter on Psychosomatic Disorders, and under the heading of Schizophrenia.

5. Phobias

Although a common condition in early childhood and adolescence, most of the phobias are of a transient nature and usually resolve themselves before maturity. Some of the most common phobias are as follows.

a Fear of animals, e.g. snakes, insects, etc.

b Fear of darkness.

c Fear of heights.

d Fear of strangers.

e Claustrophobia.

f Agoraphobia.

Most of the phobias are the result of a conditioned response. To be considered pathological, the patient will need to manifest gross disturbance of behaviour, panic attacks, and feel handicapped in sustaining everyday chores.

6. Drug and alcohol abuse

With poor licensing laws in the United Kingdom, abuse of drugs and alcohol is undoubtedly of growing concern to parents and society at large. Such activity is usually carried out in groups and quite frequently starts by some form of experimentation or curiosity.

Treatment for the disturbed adolescent is usually carried out in a specialised unit and involves a combination of behaviour therapy, individual psychotherapy and family therapy.

7. Child Abuse

Child abuse, sometimes known as 'Non-accidental injury to children', is on the increase in England and Wales. The nurse within a General hospital setting is most likely to see cases of child abuse in a casualty department or child health department. It is vital to recognise even the slightest signs and to report them immediately. This may save a life.

Causes of child abuse
a Disturbed family/home background.
b Family suffering from psychiatric disorders.
c Young and immature parents.
d Unwanted pregnancy.
e Business or financial crisis.
f One parent family.
g Persistent ill-health of the child.

Recognising the features
Although much emphasis is placed on the physical features of child abuse, it must be borne in mind that children also suffer psychological trauma through maternal/paternal deprivation, intra-psychic conflict with parents, and a feeling of non-belonging and neglect which is a direct result of non-accidental injury to children.

The visible signs are:
a Skeletal injuries.
b Burns and scalds.
c Injury to abdominal and thoracic viscera.
d Lacerations.
e Cerebral injuries.
Poisoning and incest have also been known to be associated with child abuse. In fact, sexual abuse of children is more common than has been realised. Quite often, cases are not reported to doctors or the police for fear of reprisal or even irreparable damage to the family unit.

Treatment
a Educating the parents.
b Social Services department for parental advice, and possibly to take the child into care if the home environment is not conducive to safety.
c The Children and Young Persons' Act, 1933 could be used for the child's safety.
d Educating all staff's involved.
e Public Education via the media.
f Early diagnosis as prevention.

Methods of treatment

In dealing with child and adolescent crises, the fundamental objective is to recognise the child or adolescent's needs, strivings and growth tendencies within a social and cultural background. Since most of the causes have emotional and family overtones, it is vital that an understanding is acquired of the forces that determine these conditions, and that appropriate treatment is instituted as early as possible. The following are the methods widely used by therapists in the management of child/adolescent crises.

1. Admission to a child or adolescent unit or centre.
2. Individual or group psychotherapy.
3. Family or Group Psychotherapy.
4. Meeting educational needs of the patient.
5. Use of drugs, i.e. Tranquillisers, Anti-depressants etc.
6. Play therapy.
7. Behaviour modification.
8. Psycho-drama.

Questions for discussion

1. It is often suggested that most child and adolescent crises resolve themselves by the time a person reaches adulthood. Do you agree with this statement?
2. Adolescent crises are usually the direct result of a disturbed family background. Discuss.
3. It is often quoted that the children of today are brought up in a non-disciplined environment, which therefore accounts for our sick society. Is this a fair statement?
4. Discuss the values of the treatment used by therapists in the management of child and adolescent disorders.
5. Discuss the advantages and disadvantages of nursing an adolescent in an adult psychiatric ward.

7 DRUG DEPENDENCE

Drug dependence has now become a problem of increasing concern to the medical world and to society. In clinical areas, managing such problems is viewed by nursing staff with unease and pessimism. Drug dependent patients are not solely confined to psychiatric hospitals; very often they may gain admission to casualty departments, medical/surgical wards and out-patient clinics. Such a subject is complex and, for this reason, a special chapter is devoted to it. It is intended that nurses will develop some insight into its causation and overall management in order to be better equipped to deal with casualties when such situations arise. For space reasons, this chapter is only a brief summary, and nurses wishing to develop their interest in this field will require further reading.

The objectives of this section are:
1. To define drug dependency, using W.H.O. definitions.
2. To list the possible causes of drug dependency.
3. To describe the common drugs of addiction and their effects.
4. To outline the treatment used in the management of patients suffering from drug addiction.

World Health Organisation definition

The World Health Organisation's Committee, known as the 'Expert Committee on Drugs liable to produce Addiction' defines drug addiction as follows.

'Drug addiction is a state of periodic or chronic intoxication detrimental to the individual and to society, produced by the repeated consumption of a drug (natural or synthetic.) Its characteristics include:

1. An overpowering desire or need (compulsion) to continue taking the drug and to obtain it by any means.
2. A tendency to increase the dose.
3. A psychic (psychological) and sometimes a physical dependence on the effects of the drug.

Other terms related to drug addiction which are of educational value to the nurse are the following:

1. **Habituation:** or habit-forming, is defined as a psychological dependence on the use of a drug because of the relief from tension and emotional discomfort.
2. **Physical dependence:** refers to an altered physiological state brought about by repeated administration of a drug.
3. **Tolerance:** implies a declining effect of the same dose of a drug when it is administered repeatedly over a period of time.

Aetiology

Drug addiction is a complex social problem. From this statement it is obvious that the root cause of drug dependency is sociological in nature. However, there are other, equally important, factors which either precipitate or pre-dispose to the development of drug dependency.

1. Personality disorder — sociopathy.
2. Neurotic and psychotic patients.
3. Curiosity — a search for thrills, and of expanding perceptual senses.
4. Physical illness; terminal cases.
5. 'Over-prescribing' by G.P.s.
6. A desire to belong to a peer group.
7. Social and cultural factors.

Personality

Addicts show a whole range of personality characteristics, from the normal to the neurotic, psychopathic, psychotic and sexually deviant. Although many addicts show marked personality disorders with emotional instability, immaturity and impulsiveness, these traits are also quite common in non-addicts. Behavioural changes during the process of drug taking are also of importance to the nurse. There is a decline of efficiency and reliability, the need for deception and a compulsion to obtain drugs by every possible available means.

Drugs of Addiction

1. Opiates

Heroin and morphine come into this category. Heroin is from two to ten times as potent as Morphine and is a synthetic alkeloid form of Morphine. Tolerance to the euphoric effects of the drug rapidly develops, so the user must ingest larger quantities to get his kicks. Morphine is widely used by addicts particularly when Heroin is difficult to obtain. It is either injected as a liquid or taken internally. It acts on the central nervous system as an analgesic or pain killer.

Dangers include withdrawal symptoms, e.g. sweating, nausea, vomiting, cramps, twitchings, convulsions, restlessness, agitation, tremor, yawning, irritability.

2. Hallucinogens

Drugs that alter sensory perceptions, e.g.

  a Lysergic acid diethylamide (L.S.D.)
  b Psilocybin (Sacred mushroom/God's Flesh)
  c Mescaline
  d Marijuana (Cannabis Sativa)

The abuse of Hallucinogens probably achieved its peak in the 1960s. It has been openly and irresponsibly exposed for alleged mind expanding, but prolonged use of Hallucinogens may cause cognitive dysfunction, nervous breakdowns and violence. Mental changes with associative behavioural disorders are also common. One of the remarkable aspects of these drugs is that only an extremely small amount is required in order to achieve the full effect (usually measured in microgrammes).

a L.S.D.

A powerful synthetic chemical which is derived from Ergot, a fungus that grows as a rust on rye, wheat or other grasses. It was first isolated in 1938 by Dr Albert Hoffman. It has been used in the past to treat patients with severe psychotic states. Today it is used mainly by 'junkies' in search of kicks, and by some scientists and medical personnel in the field of research and development. L.S.D. is generally taken orally in the form of a tablet, sugar cubes etc. It is absorbed through the stomach and intestines; L.S.D. is very rarely injected into the bloodstream.

Other slang terms are 'acid', 'cubes', '25' and 'pearly gates'.

It can produce disorientation, detachment from reality, and can lead to injury and even death.

b Psilocybin (psilocybe Mexicana)

This is extracted from a Mexican mushroom. It has similar effects to those of other hallucinogens, but is not as common as L.S.D. and Marijuana.

c Mescaline

A naturally occurring hallucinogen found in the 'buttons' of the Mexican cactus plant 'Peyote'. It was first isolated in 1896. It is almost always taken by mouth. The hallucinogenic effect of a full dose may last up to 12 hours.
Slang terms are 'Peyote' and 'Plant'.

d Marijuana (Cannabis Sativa)

Widely used today for social and recreational purposes. Its effects are a feeling of power, with distortions of time, space and body image proportions. It diminishes inhibitions, increases suggestibility and auditory sensitivity. It is mostly administered by smoking, either through a cigarette or a pipe. The cigarette is usually referred to as a 'joint'. It has no physical dependence, but through repeated use, psychological dependence may develop. The lasting effect of a marijuana 'trip' is usually from about 2 to 5 hours.

3. Amphetamines

Amphetamines act as central nervous system stimulants. They have been widely used for medical purposes in the treatment of obesity, behaviour disorders, fatigue, Parkinsonism and overdose of C.N.S. depressants. Some examples are:

a Dexidrine
b Benzedrine
c Methadrine

Amphetamines are taken as tablets, capsules and in injection form.

Dangers

Symptoms of withdrawal include apathy, suicidal risk and depression. States of restlessness and irritability are common, but the most serious complication of Amphetamines is the manifestation of Amphetamine psychosis. This is evident by restlessness, euphoria, paranoid ideas and hallucinations.

4. Barbiturates

A Barbiturate is a sedative and a hypnotic. It exerts a powerful depressant or calming action on the central nervous system. There are three different classifications of Barbiturates.

a Long-acting, slow-starting Barbiturates, e.g. luminal, phenobarbitone
b The intermediates, e.g. Butobarbitone, Amobarbitone
c The short-acting, e.g. Seconal, Nembutal

Addiction produces slowness of speech, difficulty in thinking, sluggishness, self-neglect, lack of attention and distractability. Withdrawal symptoms usually begin after 8 to 36 hours. Withdrawal manifests itself in the following characteristics:

twitching, intention tremor, nausea, vomiting, insomnia, hypo-tension, convulsions, delirium, visual disturbances and anxiety.

Management of drug addiction

When treating a patient dependent on drugs, the nursing problem is one of challenge and is quite often a protracted process. The nurse is not solely concerned with the drug issue, but with other equally important factors, e.g., lack of insight and motivation in the patient, anti-social attitudes of addicts and easy availability of drugs on the market.

Treatment
1. Admission to a specialised centre for drug-addicted patients.
2. Close observation, including withdrawal symptoms, T.P.R., B.P., fluid-balance, blood tests, physical examination etc.
3. Group psychotherapy, preferably with a homogenous group.
4. Occupational and recreational therapy.
5. Rehabilitation and after-care.
6. Family therapy.

Prevention
1. Health education — use of the media in providing information about drugs and their dangers.
2. Early detection is essential.
3. Medical intervention in order to reduce the ad hoc measure of prescribing drugs by doctors.
4. Legal aspects — to include severe penalties for drug 'pushers'.
5. Research into drug dependency.

Questions for discussion

1. Drug dependency is a direct result of a sick society. Discuss.
2. Self-discipline and motivation is a key factor in the management of drug addicts. How far do you agree with this statement?
3. Discuss the possible psychological and physical complications of drugs of addiction.
4. What, in your opinion, are the most successful forms of therapy for the drug addict, and why?
5. The problems of drug addiction are here to stay. Is this a reasonable statement?

Alcoholism

Consumption of alcohol has been, to a large extent, an acceptable norm of Western society. In France, for instance, drinking of wine is a way of life. Alcoholism is an illness; and like any other illness, it has definable aetiology and clinical manifestations. It therefore requires treatment, preferably in a Unit which caters solely for the needs of the alcoholic.

The objectives of this section are:
1. To define the term 'Alcoholism'.
2. To describe its underlying causes.

3. To discuss the stages and degrees of alcoholism.
4. To list the social, physical and psychiatric complications of alcoholism.
5. To outline briefly its treatment.

Definition (W.H.O.)

The World Health Organisation defines alcoholism as, 'those excessive drinkers whose dependence upon alcohol has attained such a degree that they show a noticeable mental disturbance or an interference with their bodily or mental health, their inter-personal relations and their smooth social and economic functioning, or who show the prodromal signs of such development. They therefore require treatment'.

On a national scale, the problem is probably more underrated, as much covering-up is done by the family and the patient himself and his friends. It is estimated that there are almost a million alcoholics in the British Isles — 2% of the population, more common than Schizophrenia. The number is forever increasing.

Causes of Alcoholism

Alcohol is condoned by the public on the premise that it satisfies some intense psychological need. To some it gives courage, to others confidence and the provision of companionship. The primary cause of alcoholism is based on the Freudian theory of oral fixation. Other underlying causes are, to a large extent, of a secondary nature, e.g.
1. Social and professional.
2. Personality disorders, usually sociopathic.
3. Neurotic disorders.
4. Physical illness.
5. Major psychoses.
Family histories demonstrate that alcoholics usually come from broken homes with an over-indulgent and over-protective parent. The psychodynamic of the family is obviously an area in which the therapist is interested.

Social and cultural factors influence the amount of alcoholism. Drinking among the Jews and Chinese is less frequent than among the races of Europe and the United States.

Properties of Alcohol

It is generally agreed that alcohol is a depressant and not a stimulant and that it reduces both mental and muscular efficiency. It acts as an anaesthetic on the central nervous system, starting on the higher centres and gradually progressing downwards. Thus, its first effects are to remove inhibitions, impair motor control and lower the level of awareness. Higher levels cause a lack of control of speech, difficulty in walking and finally even a lowered level of consciousness, with coma and eventual death. In an advanced stage of intoxication, it is more common for a person to die through inhaling vomit than from the effects of alcohol itself.

Stages in Alcoholism
Alcoholics usually follow sequential phases in their illness. Prognosis is good at its earliest onset, but gradually becomes poor, especially in the chronic phase. The four phases in alcoholism are universally acknowledged:

Pre-Alcoholic Symptomatic Phase
Here, the individual starts drinking on a social basis, but he soon realises that alcohol provides relief for his psychological difficulties. Further tensions, anxieties and frustrations lead to alcohol more frequently. The drinking becomes heavier in the evening.

The Prodromal Phase
At this stage, normal activities are carried out without repercussion, although the individual's consumption of alcohol is on the increase. Denial is common, and amnesia from the previous night's drinking is also a feature. He may start drinking secretly and develop guilty feelings about his drinking. This phase may last anything from six months to five years.

The Crucial Phase
The main feature of this phase is loss of control, to the point where the drinker cannot stop as long as he is able, by any means, to obtain more. He becomes a solitary drinker, who hoards bottles because he fears being without alcohol, and he probably finds that he cannot start the day without a drink. Social and personality deterioration occur at this stage. He suffers from tremor, cramps and a craving if he is deprived of alcohol. Aggression and persistent remorse become a feature. He becomes self-centred, loses outside interests, and neglects food and personal hygiene.

The Chronic Phase
In this phase, drinking is incessant, gradually increasing in quantity to a point of complete intoxication. There is also marked ethical deterioration and impairment of the cognitive process. Physical and psychiatric complications are evident at this stage.

Complications of Alcoholism

a *Social*
1. Unhappy marriage and divorce.
2. Housing problems.
3. Job loss.
4. Financial difficulties.
5. Loss of friends.
6. Loss of status.
7. Social isolation.

b *Physical*
1. Gastritis — 25% of patients attending gastro-enterological clinics are alcoholics; 10% of admissions to a general hospital are alcoholics.
2. Peripheral Neuritis — due to lack of Vitamin B.
3. Cirrhosis of the liver — 65% of patients with this complaint are alcoholics.
4. Epilepsy — common at various stages of alcoholism.
5. Delirium Tremens — 'the shakes'.
6. Coma — which may lead to death.
7. Congenital abnormalities — caused by heavy drinking during the first three months of pregnancy.
8. Other complications include Acute and Chronic Pancreatitis, cardiac disorders and Malabsorption Syndrome.

c *Psychiatric*
1. Anxiety states.
2. Depressive symptoms as a result of guilt or remorse.
3. Suicide.
4. Pathological jealousy of their sexual partners.
5. Alcoholic Dementia.
6. Alcoholic Paranoia.
7. Korsakoff's Psychosis — characterised by amnesia, confabulation and marked suggestability, together with peripheral neuritis.
8. Wernicke's Encephalopathy.
9. Alcoholic Hallucinosis.

Treatment of Alcoholism

As stated before, prognosis is poor. Even with intensive treatment, relapses are inevitable. Motivation and insight are potent determinants of a sustained recovery.
1. Acknowledgement of the problem.

2. Use of Antabuse (Disulfram) and Abstem (Citrated Calcium Carbimide)
3. Aversion therapy.
4. Group psychotherapy — preferably with homogenous groups.
5. Use of 'drying-out' centres and hostels.
6. Educating the public in normal drinking.
7. Follow-up is essential.
8. Alcoholics Anonymous.
9. Family and marital therapy, to be used in conjunction with other therapies.

Questions for Discussion
1. 'Alcoholism is endemic in Western society.' Discuss this statement.
2. Discuss the psychosocial and physical implications of alcoholic indulgence. Support your answer with statistical evidence.
3. Argue the statement that 'Alcoholics are best treated within a therapeutic community milieu'.
4. Discuss the part played by personality in the development of alcoholism.
5. 'The majority of alcoholics are involved with the Law'. Could you justify this statement in the light of your own clinical experience?
6. Discuss the psychoanalytical theory of oral fixation as a causative factor in alcoholism.
7. It is claimed that Group Psychotherapy is a most effective tool in the management of alcoholic patients. How far do you agree with this statement?
8. Why do people consume alcohol?
9. Many patients with alcohol problems do not require admission to hospital. What alternative methods of care are available?

8 PSYCHOSOMATIC DISORDERS

Psychosomatic medicine plays an important part in the field of mental health. Hence, because of its co-existence with physical illness, it serves of immense value to general nurses practising within the field of general nursing. Psychiatric disorders are notably frequent in casualty departments, in medical wards, in dermatological units and gynaecological and gastro-enterological clinics. All physical illnesses have psychological effects, a few have psychological causes.

The objectives of this section are:
a To introduce the concept of psychosomatic medicine as a possible instrument in understanding physical illnesses.
b To describe, using the bodily systems, the causes, psychiatric manifestations and treatment of psychosomatic illnesses.

Psychosomatic medicine deals with several groups of patients. Physical illness, no matter what form it takes, evokes some degree of anxiety and stress. These psychological phenomena are potentially destructive elements, and the nurse in the general field must be skilled at recognising these features. Failing to recognise them may result in prolonged hospitalisation and delayed recovery.

There are three groups of patients which may be considered under the term of psychosomatic medicine:
1. Those who suffer from various physical symptoms, but who do not have a bodily disease that may serve as a cause for the symptoms. As a result of failing to recognise that such disorders have emotional origin, physicians have often labelled these conditions as 'functional' or 'organic' in origin.
2. Those where a physical disease exists, but the causative factors are of an emotional nature.
3. Those where the patient does have actual organic disease but where certain of his symptoms arise not from the disease process but as a result of psychological phenomena.

It is vital that the physician undertakes a thorough physical and psychological examination of the patient, and does not confine his examination to the seeking of a diagnosis on a physical/organic basis. Unless he does so, he may overlook any psychosomatic components in organic disease, and therefore make treatment difficult.

Causes of Psychosomatic Disorders

It is difficult to pinpoint an exact cause for the development of psychosomatic conditions. A list of pre-disposing causes follows:
1. Stress may precipitate psychosomatic illness.
2. Heredity.
3. Repressed emotional conflict.

Psychophysiological Reactions

It is easy to describe the psychosomatic conditions from a standpoint of classification into the various bodily systems

1. Cardiovascular System

It is assumed generally that stress induces emotional change and contributes to the development of Myocardial Infarction, Coronary Artery diseases and Angina Pectoris. In a study by Roserman and Friedman, a group of middle-aged men was selected for their behaviour patterns of great drive, competitiveness and a sense of urgency which derived from their commitment to holding top executive jobs. That such a group was chosen as representing those most at risk from cardio-vascular disorders is significant, and the significance has been confirmed over and over again.

Hypertension

The primary cause is emotional tension operating within the central nervous system causing wide-spread vaso-constriction. Many hypertensives are neurotic and have compulsive and perfectionist characteristics in their personalities.

Treatment
1. Use of hypotensive drugs.
2. Psychotherapy.

Migraine

Aetiology — most sufferers are usually ambitious and conform to strict behaviour patterns. Hostility to siblings and other family members is common. There usually exists a history of migraine in the family.

Treatment
1. Use of analgesics may help.
2. Psychotherapy is recommended.
3. Social therapy to sublimate aggressive drives may also help.

2. Musculo-Skeletal System

Rheumatoid Arthritis

Patients suffering from rheumatoid arthritis are usually described as being well adapted to new situations, rather introverted, but active physically and intellectually. Sudden death in the family, separation or rejection, the birth of a child, miscarriage or disappointment may trigger off an attack.

Treatment
1. Use of analgesics.
2. Use of cortisone derivatives.
3. Psychotherapy is effective if given over a long period of time.

3. Endocrine System

Two main psychosomatic conditions in this category are:
1. Thyrotoxicosis.
2. Diabetes Mellitus.

Thyrotoxicosis

This condition arises largely in sensitive persons who manifest a marked feeling of insecurity and are lacking in responsibility. There is usually a long-standing history of emotional turmoil and psychological maladjustment. Apart from physical manifestations of the condition, there are also concommittant features of overactivity, emotional instability, depression, agitation, and, in some cases, a psychotic reaction may develop.

Treatment
1. Use of anti-thyroid drugs.
2. Use of tranquillisers.
3. Psychotherapy is essential.

Diabetes Mellitus

The condition is often associated with periods of severe emotional stress; the patients usually have passive and immature characteristics to their personalities in the search for affection and attention. A sudden psychological trauma, e.g. rejection, death of a loved one, may produce this condition.

Treatment
1. Use of insulin.
2. Dietary regime.
3. Psychotherapy.

4. Skin

It is one of the obvious and common areas affected. Dermatologists place great emphasis on psychological factors in the development of skin conditions, such as Pruritis, Hyperhidrosis, Neuro-dermatitis, Eczema and Psoriasis. It is claimed that the more severe the emotional stress, the greater the affliction to the skin.

5. Genito-Urinary System

There is a close anatomical relationship between the sexual organs and the exretory system. Parental attitudes towards toilet training (urination and defecation) and society's view of human sexuality and behaviour poses great emotional stress to the developing individual. In man, the most common psychosomatic symptoms are premature ejaculation and impotence, whereas in the female frigidity, dysmenorrhoea, premenstrual tension and dyspareunia are the common expressions of psychopathology.

6. Alimentary System

Food is often associated with emotion; lack of or deprivaton of food usually results in feelings of tension. A sense of relief and joy is often displayed when a hungry baby is given food. Psychosomatic disturbances of the alimentary system are common, e.g. Peptic Ulcer, Ulcerative Colitis, Obesity, Anorexia Nervosa are but a few.

Peptic Ulcer

Psychogenic factors are of importance in the aetiology of Peptic Ulcer. There is striking scientific evidence to support such a claim. Predisposing factors are:
1. Genetic.
2. Hyperchlohydria, common in peptic ulcer, is claimed to be due to an increase in hydrochloric acid in anxious and stressful patients as a result of inner conflict.
3. A higher level of Uropepsin in the stool and urine.

Treatment
1. Medical — **a** use of antacids/alkali drugs
    b dietary control.
2. Surgical — partial or complete gastrectomy.
3. Psychotherapeutic — prolonged psychoanalysis, with possibly a change of job and environment.

Ulcerative Colitis
Precipitating factors are:
1. Bereavement.
2. Romantic disharmony.
3. Loss of a part of the body.
4. Changes in psychological status.
5. Loneliness.
6. Diminished self-esteem.
7. Academic work failures.

Treatment
1. Treatment is usually carried out by a physician, but the psychiatrist's contribution is normally aimed at emotional security and the establishment of a solid, dependant relationship with the patient.
2. Regressive therapy is also a useful therapeutic tool for the psychiatrist.
3. Intensive psychotherapy.
4. Medical treatment may involve the use of antibiotics and the use of cortisone enemas.
5. In severe cases, a partial colectomy with a colostomy may be performed.

Obesity
It is often suggested that food is a substitute for love and affection, and that obesity is a result of deprived affection. To some extent this is true, as we frequently see depressed patients resorting to food in search of comfort and reassurance. Recent research has revealed that the hypothalamic areas in the brain may play a large part in our eating habits. Certain specific brain lesions in the hypothalamus may result in hyperphagia without an actual increase in hunger.

Family psychodynamics are often the predisposing cause of obesity in children. The mother is usually the dominant family member, is over-protective and has high expectations of achievement for the child. In many instances, the obese child is not a wanted child.

Being obese has its advantages. It often represents the desire to be strong and powerful. The child, especially in a social environment, is conspicuous and may receive attention through this source.

Treatment
1. Successful treatment of the obese person requires the knowledge of his total personality.
2. Psychotherapy — preferably family psychotherapy if a child is involved.

3. Behaviour modification with the use of positive reinforcement.
4. Exercise coupled with a controlled diet.

Anorexia Nervosa
A psychosomatic disorder first described by Sir William Guss in 1868 and given the name Anorexia Nervosa in 1874. Anorexics are usually common in females, but males have been known to develop this condition.

Personality traits
Most patients are intellectually superior, and are introverted, stubborn, selfish, perfectionistic, and at times manipulative. There also exists a drive for punishment and thinness.

Clinical features
1. Loss of appetite.
2. Low metabolic rate ($\downarrow$ BMR).
3. Dryness of skin.
4. Agitation.
5. Constipation.
6. Falling out of hair.
7. Amenorrhoea.

Aetiology
1. Cosmetic — a strong desire to be slim — highly influenced by the media.
2. Mother/daughter or father/son conflict.
3. Sibling rivalry and jealousy.
4. Over-protectiveness.
5. Frustration in heterosexual adjustments.
6. Pregnancy fantasy may initiate a patient to diet.

Treatment
1. Medical — to preserve life in severe cases by feeding until a desired weight is established.
2. Psychological — the establishment of a supportive, encouraging, therapeutic relationship with the patient. Use of insight therapy and family psychotherapy are essential to achieve a reasonable degree of success.
3. Token economy.
4. Modified insulin therapy to promote weight gain.
5. Constant observation and supervision is needed.

7. Respiratory System

Certain emotional expressions such as crying or laughter bring about a physiological change in respiration. Anger quite often leads to hyperventilation syndrome.

Hyperventilation Syndrome

This condition is often induced by fear or anger. The common complaints are usually of lightheadedness or giddiness, an increase in the depth and rapidity of respiration, a feeling of faintness, profuse perspiration, feelings of pressure in the thorax and disturbed sensations in the fingertips or toes. Hyperventilation syndrome may also be caused by febrile conditions, anoxemia and high external temperatures.

Treatment
In most cases, it is recommended that patients receive psychotherapy.

Asthma

Asthmatic attack is no longer solely associated with a specific antigen. More and more cases reveal a strong emotional predisposition in an event of an attack, e.g. bereavement, business reverses, academic failures, etc. The asthmatic personality is often irritable, lacking in confidence, submissive and anxious. The patient usually has a clinging personality and is to a large extent very dependant on his parents.

Treatment
1. Medical — urgent attention is required in treating the actual attack by medical means.
2. Psychological — psychotherapy is effective in bringing about relief to this condition. In cases where children are involved, family psychotherapy may be recommended.

Most patients with psychosomatic conditions require long-term psychotherapy, and, in some instances, psychoanalysis. When children are involved and the psychopathology is the family, then family psychotherapy is highly recommended. Properly structured psychotherapeutic sessions with the client may reduce the possibility of relapse in later years.

Practice Questions

1. Define psychosomatic illness.
2. List the main physical symptoms of the body and indicate for each a psychosomatic condition which may affect it.
3. There are some disorders which may be termed Somatopsychic,

i.e. physical illnesses resulting in psychiatric or psychological disturbances. Give two examples.

4. What is hyperphagia?

5. Can boys suffer from Anorexia Nervosa?

6. From your reading of the chapter on Psychosomatic Illness do you gain the impression that generally patients suffering from these conditions are of lower social status and rather unintelligent, or of higher status and bright?

7. Would you say that in the causation of Asthma, allergens are:
   a a direct cause
   b a predisposing cause, or
   c a precipitating cause?

8. In studies it has been found that more bus drivers suffer from Coronary Infarction than bus conductors. What may account for this?

9. What do you understand by intra-psychic conflict? Give two examples.

10. Give two examples of skin manifestations of stress or emotion.

11. 'Bodily diseases always affect mind function'. Is this a reasonable statement?

12. 'Pregnancy is a self-induced psychosomatic condition'. First justify this statement, then criticise it.

Answers

1. One definition might be: 'those disorders which show physical manifestations where the cause, or a significant component of it, is psychological'.
2. Cardiovascular — coronary infarction.
   Skeletal — rheumatoid arthritis.
   Respiratory — asthma.
   Digestive — duodenal ulcer.
   Endocrine — thyrotoxicosis.
   Reproductive — impotence.
   Urinary — enuresis.
3. Gout, resulting in irrascible temper.
   Influenza, resulting in post-influenzal depression.
4. Overeating, with or without great appetite.
5. Yes, but only very rarely.
6. Generally such patients are intelligent and of Social Classes 1, 2 and 3, i.e. middle to high.
7. The evidence is that allergens are precipitatory in the causation of asthma.
8. Some factors which may be considered are that bus drivers have a job which is:
   a continually stressful in coping with (especially) city traffic.
   b responsible for public safety.
   c sedentary; little exercise possible.
   d unremitting; no 'mini-breaks' possible while driving.
   Compare with the role of the bus conductor.
9. Intra-psychic conflict is where choices of perceived equal merit have to be made. Such conflict may occur in a family torn between sending an aged relative into a nursing home, or managing the relative at home. Another example may occur when one is torn between a job which is disliked, but is well-paid, and a job which is congenial but poorly-paid.
10. Blushing, pallor (white with anger), goose-flesh, skin 'crawling' with horror or disgust, hair standing on end.
11. Yes, on the whole. We talk of a sick person being 'not himself today'. Most illnesses make one feel miserable, self-centred and demanding. Others reject company and seek isolation.
12. There is no right answer to this question. Suffice it to say that there are people who hold such an opinion, others who do not and neither group is wrong.

9 TREATMENT AND NURSING CARE

The aim of this chapter is to provide a brief introduction to some of the multitudinous forms of treatment of the mentally ill, together with some hints on nursing the patient with some of the more common conditions. Notes are appended on the Mental Health Act 1983.

The objectives, then, are to present:

a A short philosophy of care, with particular reference to the 'nursing process'.

b A precis of four important methods of treatment under the heading of 'Physical treatments'.

c Some indication of the more common forms of therapeutic activities in which nurses are involved.

d Useful hints in the nursing management of some of the more frequently met conditions.

e Guidance on the approach to patients expected of a nurse.

f A flow-chart outlining the stages of progression from admission to rehabilitation and discharge.

g An abbreviated form of the main provisions of recent legislation.

Nursing the psychiatric patient

In the days when our mental hospitals were founded, little treatment was available for the psychiatric patient, and the public were anxious to see that the mentally ill were locked up in institutions well away from the public view. During the past few years a change, tantamount to a revolution, has been going on, and is accelerating. This change has been effected not only by scientific progress, but also by a new dynamism among those who care for the mentally ill. Better education and training has resulted in higher professional standards of care practised by nurses and other para-medical staff.

The stigma of mental illness is declining as the public becomes better informed, and it is slowly becoming realised that the majority of mentally ill patients will never enter a psychiatric hospital for in-patient treatment. Of those that do, the vast majority are admitted on an informal basis, with the same rights as those physically ill patients admitted to a general hospital. Much active psychiatry is practised in out-patient clinics, and many patients are treated at home by their own general practitioners. Many organisations, voluntary and statutory, assist in the task of keeping people out of hospital and functioning normally in society. There are day-hospitals and night-hospitals, day-care centres, 'half-way hostels', sheltered workshops, rehabilitation centres, community clubs, clinics and recreational centres. Virtually every health district has its Community Psychiatric Nurses (CPNs), taking their skills into patients' homes and commonly supporting more mentally ill patients thereby than are found in local psychiatric hospitals.

The general nurse is well used to treating patients with fractures, inflamed gall-bladders and coronary occlusions; seeing patients from the onset of their disorders to (hopefully) cure and discharge. She may feel confident that she knows what disease is all about, having witnessed it through all its stages. She will (or should) be less confident about medical disorders, since the hospital nurse sees the patient only for a limited period, and realises that in most cases the patient has suffered his disorder for months or years before coming into hospital. When the patient is discharged from the medical ward, the nurse may be well aware that his disorder is not cured. Stabilised, contained, improved perhaps, but 'cures' are rarely spoken of in general medicine. The community Nurse and the Health Visitor have another tale to tell . . .

Psychiatric illness is very similar. The psychiatric nurse working in a hospital commonly sees the patient only during the brief hospital interlude, but the disorder may well be life-long.

In the general hospital, efforts are made to treat the whole person, not just his disease, as it is realised that a person's needs extend well beyond his need to be rid of his clinical condition. Individualised care planning, incorporating 'activities of daily living' on the lines of the so-called 'Nursing Process' have been introduced into the majority of the general wards. This has been a major step in providing comprehensive care, and is resulting in nurses becoming as socially aware as they are clinically aware. The goodwill and professionalism of nurses practising such forms of holistic care is however thwarted by the short period of in-patient stay so common in, especially, the surgical wards. For the patient, his over-riding need is to have his clinical condition attended to, and for the short period of his stay he can suppress his other less-demanding needs on a 'let's tackle one thing at a time' basis. Indeed, he may actively resent any nursing intrusion into his life. Well able to cope and fend for his family and himself when he is physically well, he requires only 100% of medical and nursing care directed solely at his disorder. If his hospital stay is extended, as in orthopaedic wards for example, the situation is different, and the whole panoply of the Nursing Process can be brought to bear.

The patient in the psychiatric hospital is commonly there for much longer, from 4 weeks to years, even a lifetime. His home, work, recreation and friends are all in the hospital, in many cases. Further, the condition which brought him into hospital in the first place is largely a social one. Schizophrenia, for example, is not life-threatening, physically painful nor prostrating; *socially*, however, it is devastating. The whole of his care may be aimed at social reintegration only, once the immediate signs and symptoms have subsided. Working with the psychiatrically ill requires a different approach: an all-embracing holistic approach to care. Happily, we usually have more time at our disposal to attend to the patient's non-clinical needs. It would be, however, too easy (and too clinical?) to divide his needs into two distinct and separate areas, clinical and non-clinical, since many non-clinical activities (occupation, recreation, etc.) can be highly therapeutic. Remembering the social nature of his disorder, such non-clinical activities may be more therapeutic than if his disease were merely treated as a clinical entity.

No authority can detail the nursing care required for any particular patient, general or psychiatric. Everyone is wholly different, and should be treated as such; their needs, social situation, moods, finances and conditions change. Our approach must necessarily be flexible. In searching for a starting point wherewith to begin our care for any particular patient, we may take heed of the one link which groups many patients together, their clinical condition. True, this line of approach is limited, but it provides a useful starting point; individualised care can follow once we are underway.

The 'medical model' of care has been much criticised, since by itself it takes no account of the patient as a whole person, but we must not discard the baby with the bathwater; were it not for his disorder, the patient would not be in hospital, requiring any sort of care.

Physical Treatment

The use of physical treatment in psychiatry has been, from time immemorial, an issue of great controversy, both on scientific and moral grounds. There is, even today, scepticism about its real value in patients' care. However, some aspects of physical treatments have established themselves as important therapies in psychiatry.

TABLE 1.1

ANTIDEPRESSANTS	
TRICYCLICS	
Amitriptyline (Tryptizol)	50 – 100 mg.
Imipramine (Tofranil)	100 – 225 mg.
Trimipramine (Surmontil)	75 – 300 mg.
MONOAMINE OXIDASE INHIBITORS (MAOI)	
Tranylcypromine (Parnate)	20 – 30 mg.
Phenelzine (Nardil)	45 – 60 mg.
Lithium Carbonate (Priadel)	1 – 1.8 mg.
MAJOR TRANQUILLIZERS	
PHENOTHIAZINES	
Chlorpromazine (Largactil)	75 – 800 mg.
Promazine (Sparine)	50 – 800 mg.
Fluphenazine (Moditen)	1 – 15 mg.
Thioridazine (Melleril)	30 – 600 mg.
Perphenazine (Fentazin)	2 – 15 mg.
BUTRYPHENONES	
Trifluoperidol (Triperidol)	0.5 – 8 mg.
Haloperidol (Serenace)	6 – 12 mg.
MINOR TRANQUILLIZERS	
BENZODIAZEPINES	
Diazepam (Valium)	5 – 30 mg.
Chlordiazepoxide (Librium)	10 – 100 mg.
Lorazepam (Ativan)	2 – 4 mg.
CARBAMATES	
Meprobamate (Equanil)	0.4 – 1.2 mg.
OTHER TRANQUILLIZERS	
Chlormethiazole (Heminevrin)	100 – 150 mg.

Common Drugs used in Psychiatry

One of the most spectacular developments in psychiatric medicine has been the introduction, in 1952, of the phenothiazine groups of drugs for the treatment of the psychoses. Following such development, other new chemical compounds have been synthesized in the forms of Anti-depressants, Anti-convulsants and other related drugs in the management of the mentally ill. (See Table 1.1)

Tranquillisers

Phenothiazines (Major tranquillisers). Most phenothiazines cause general depression of the Central Nervous System. The common side-effects are:

Dryness of the mouth, constipation, dizziness, insomnia, blood dyscrasias, jaundice, photosensitivity, headache, drowsiness, tachycardia.

Antidepressants

Of the antidepressants, monoamine oxidase inhibitors (MAOI) take 10 to 14 days to become effective. They must not be given in conjunction with foods containing tyramines e.g. cheese, alcohol, yoghurt, meat and yeast extracts (Bovril and Marmite) and broad beans; a severe hypertensive reaction may occur. MAOIs and tricyclic drugs, must not, for the same reason, be used together.

Electro-Convulsive Therapy

History: Originating in 1933, convulsive therapy was first used by a Hungarian doctor Ladislaus von Meduna, who injected camphor in oil intramuscularly into patients to produce a convulsion. In 1938, two Italians, Cerletti and Bini, made use of electricity to produce similar reactions. Later still, short-acting anaesthetics and muscle relaxants were introduced to prevent many of the complications which occurred with E.C.T. such as bone dislocation, crush fractures, broken teeth, tongue injury and respiratory complications. Such a method is now known as Modified Electro-Convulsive Therapy. The more modern method was introduced by Lancaster et al in 1957. They described a technique of producing generalised convulsions by applying the electrodes to the non-dominant side of the brain. This is known as Unilateral Modified E.C.T., and has been adopted as standard procedure in some hospitals.

Indications for Use

1. *Depressive illnesses*
   a E.C.T. is very effective in Endogenous and Involutional Depression when these do not respond to antidepressant drugs.

   b In some selected cases of neurotic depression when anti-depressants have failed.

Psychotic disorders
   a In Schizophrenic illnesses.
   b Sometimes to control mania, but mostly used to treat depression of manic-depressive illness.
   c Puerperal psychosis.
   d Confusional states, non-organic in nature.

Contra-indications
1. *Any major physical illness*
   a Severe respiratory conditions.
   b Severe cardio-vascular disorders.
   c Severe cerebro-vascular conditions.
   d Osteoporosis, spondylosis and kyphosis.

2. *Pregnancy*
During the first four months, E.C.T. is not advisable.

3. *Anxiety states*

Precautionary measures
1. Thorough physical examination.
2. Chest X-Ray.
3. Electro-cardiograph (E.C.G.) to exclude cardiac diseases.
4. Possible dental examination.

Method
1. Takes place in E.C.T room.
2. Proper psychological preparation of the patient is essential.
3. Atropine sulphate 0.6 mg is given 45 to 60 minutes before treatment.
4. Sodium Thiopentone (Pentothal 200–500 mgs) or Brietal Sodium (5 to 10 ml) is given, depending on age and weight of the patient.
5. After the patient has been anaesthetised, muscle relaxation is given, i.e. Scoline 0.6 to 1 ml.
6. Convulsion is induced by the introduction of electric current via saline-moistened electrodes across the temples.
   a Bilateral method. The electrodes are placed 5 cm above the mid-point of a line drawn from the lateral angle of the eye to the external auditory meatus.
   b Unilateral method. The non-dominant side is selected. One electrode is applied to the temporal region, 4 cm above the mid-point

of the ear-eye line and the other is placed above the ear over the parietal region, 6 cm from the first electrode.

Post-electro-convulsive therapy convulsion
1. Impairment of recent memory normally occurs with bilateral E.C.T. Only slight impairment is noticed with unilateral E.C.T.
2. The complications may include drowsiness, breathing difficulties, laryngitis and scoline apnoea.

Psychosurgery

The operation lobectomy, sometimes also known as lobotomy, was performed widely in the late 1940s in the treatment of anxiety states, tension, disorganised behaviour, depression and obsessional symptoms. Although the results were satisfactory, the complications outweighed the benefits, notably serious personality changes, cerebral infections and, in some cases, convulsions.

Techniques of Lobectomy
A surgical procedure consisting of severing the connection of fibres between the thalamus and the frontal lobe; first developed by a Portuguese neurologist, Egas Moniz and first performed by the neuro-surgeon Almeida Lima in 1935.

Indications for use
Best results occur for the following conditions:
1. Tension
2. Stress
3. Depression
4. Phobias
5. Obsessional/Compulsive neurosis
6. Aggression
7. Hallucinatory and delusional experiences
The results are favourable in patients who are operated upon when all other alternatives have failed. In some cases, recovery is dramatic. Having said that, there is still a great danger of cerebral infection, permanent brain damage and personality and behavioural changes, and such surgery is only used as a last resort in intolerable conditions.

Nursing and Treating the Psychiatric Patient in Hospital

The clear-cut distinctions between the role of the nurse in the general hospital and her medical and para-medical colleagues are not parelleled in the psychiatric hospital to the same extent. The psychiatric nurse acts as a link between the other hospital professionals, and her work frequently overlaps that of her colleagues:

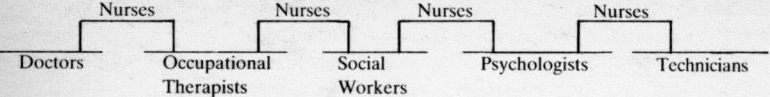

Some of the methods and features of this multi-professional approach to care are outlined below.

Therapeutic Community The ward or unit staff, from the consultant psychiatrist to the ward domestic, aim collectively to provide an environment conducive to the patient's recovery. All have a right and an obligation to contribute their views and ideas to maintaining an encouraging atmosphere wherein patients can rehabilitate themselves by initiating activity and making decisions.

Case Conference On a regular basis the multi-professional team, together with learners from the various disciplines, meet to discuss individual patients. Contributions are invited from everyone, in the form of advice, observations and suggestions, in order to achieve consistency of effort and consensus agreement about the direction that care should follow.

Behaviour Therapy Very useful in treating phobic and anxiety states in patients, the treatment is based upon learning theories, and aims at deconditioning or desensitizing them in situations previously considered by the patient to be threatening, frightening or distasteful. Ever-increasing 'doses' of the fear-provoking stimuli are gradually introduced to the patient by, generally, one therapist who is commonly a nurse. Trust in, and an unshakeable rapport with the nurse is paramount.

Individual Psychotherapy On a one-to-one basis, patients are talked through their problems and offered support, sympathy, understanding, acceptance and an outlet for suppressed fears and misgivings. Advice is usually sought by the patient; giving it is rarely as effective as counselling, wherein patients are supported in the analysis of their own problems and are encouraged to formulate a plan conducive to recovery and to maintain it subsequently.

Group Psychotherapy This may be 'analytical' or 'supportive' in character, for neurotic and psychotic patients respectively. It is rarely wise to mix both kinds of patients in group psychotherapy. Groups are variable in size, the larger groups tend to be 'open', with staff and patients coming and going without disturbing the informal free-for-all discussions taking place. Closed groups are smaller, more formal, intensive and barred to outsiders, be they staff or patients. Analytical groups seek to interpret problems and seek, through the medium of others' observations, to find how one's behaviour may influence the occurrence of these problems. Supportive groups encourage 'good' and positive behaviour and point out the effects of 'bad' and negative behaviour. Pressure from other patients in all groups ('peer pressure') is often more efficacious than staff pressure in bringing about therapeutic changes.

Family and Marital Therapy The patient's wife/husband may be invited to participate in psychotherapeutic sessions with the patient if he/she can contribute or if it is apparent that the marriage partner is involved in the causation of the disorder. Similarly, other family members, or even whole families, may be invited. Such sessions are almost always, necessarily, 'closed' events.

Aversion By associating an unpleasant stimulus with what was previously a pleasurable activity, an aversion is induced. Drug-induced vomiting following the drinking of alcohol may be effective in treating alcoholism. Drug-taking and various sexual perversions may be averted by associating them with electric shocks. Supportive psychotherapy is an essential adjunct to these aversion sessions. There is usually one major proviso before commencing a series of aversion treatments: the patient must want to be cured.

In the day-to-day nursing of the psychiatrically ill patient, the general rules of treatment apply: treat the signs and symptoms, then remove the cause. In psychiatry, the former is usually easier than the latter. In treating the patient symptomatically, such is the enormous diversity of psychiatric signs and symptoms, only a few broad hints can be given.

Depression A bright, cheerful environment is conducive to lifting the patient's mood, together with convivial company and not too demanding activity. Certainly in neurotic (exogenous) depression, these may have a very beneficial effect. In psychotic (endogenous) depression, the patient may not, however, be helped by such measures, nor will he change by being forced into unwanted activity.

Dances, parties and discos may be just the thing for many people, but remember, for a substantial number of perfectly normal and healthy people, parties and discos are anathema. Such people, when depressed, would find such events horrendous. With patients in misery, bordering on depressive stupor, even communicating with staff is impossible. Such patients desperately need the warmth of human contact, but cannot establish it themselves. Holding the patient's hand, or an arm around his shoulders, may say more to a patient unable to talk than all the 'Cheer up's, 'Never mind's and other useless platitudes put together.

Mania Ensure, however difficult it may be, that the patient eats sufficiently. Seemingly his boundless energy is expended on everything but eating. Often, he would be better served at a table on his own than with a group of other patients. A patient in mania is often irritable and irritating; he must be protected from the wrath of other patients, and they from him. Providing this two-way protection may tax the resources of the staff sorely, but must be attempted. Jobs given to this patient should be plentiful and able to be quickly done; his attention span is very limited, and longer, more demanding tasks will frequently be left unfinished.

Delusions These are false beliefs with no foundation. They may exist in a Schizophrenic patient as a simple 'wrong idea', or as a systematised delusional state wherein the patient's beliefs are surrounded by highly complex reasons and explanations of the 'rightness' of his belief.

The nurse, after initial trials to change the patient's mind, soon learns a hard lesson, i.e., you cannot argue with a delusion. Every nurse tries, every nurse fails. If a patient mentions a delusion, change the subject at once and do not refer to it again. Humouring the patient by a pretended belief in his idea only makes it worse — it reinforces his idea that the subject of his belief is true.

Hallucinations These are false perceptions with no outside stimulus to cause them. 'Talking to oneself' is not a sign of anything except normality. The schizophrenic patient does not talk to himself, he talks to his 'voices'.

Again, the rule is to distract the patient's attention onto something which is real, and which is also perceived by the patient to be real.

Apathy Arguably the greatest problem faced by the nurse in the psychiatric hospital. It is often thought by the general nurse that violence is a major feature encountered in psychiatric hospitals. Far from it; violence is a rarity, largely because the psychiatric nurse is a past-master at preventing it. Once it occurs, however, the psychiatric nurse is generally no more skilled in dealing with it than her general colleagues.

Apathy is in a different league. It is ever-present in the wards, and is a destructive force leading to institutionalisation. The resources of many professionals in the Occupational Therapy, Industrial Therapy and Recreational Therapy departments are stretched in all hospitals to combat the insidious menace of apathy among patients. A concerted, consistent and continuous effort must be made by all staff, especially the nurse to utilise every facility the hospital possesses, and which she personally possesses, to combat it.

Establishing satisfactory rapport

A nurse must be prepared for anything when admitting a mentally sick person and be constantly on her guard. She must be **observant**, for states of neuroses are not always clear-cut and the patient may present symptoms of various mental reactions.

Nurse's Personality

One important thing to realize is that **personality** plays a large part in the nursing of these patients, and a nurse must recognise when she is unable to help the patient and be willing to say so. Certain patients respond best to the quiet, unobtrusive nurse, some feel more comfortable when they are guided by a self-sufficient, motherly type and others are more responsive to the nurse who is the enthusiastic leader type.

Other Important Factors

Apart from recognising your type of personality, there are other qualities in a nurse which facilitate an agreeable relationship, especially with mentally ill patients.

Cheerfulness: The greatest asset. Smile — encouragement. Happy and content in adversity.

Politeness: Polite, from the Latin word meaning 'polish', indicates culture. A nurse must strive always to be polite.

Tactfulness: The word 'tact' means touch. It may be interpreted as skill in handling a situation.

Friendliness: This may be interpreted as a warm feeling reaching out to the other person; it embraces politeness, confidence and hospitality.

Patience: A nurse must possess or cultivate this virtue.

Truthfulness: Much more essential for a nurse to be truthful than to demand it in a patient.

Even Temper: This is a great asset when dealing with people who are emotionally upset. Unless a nurse realizes that 'emotion stirs up emotion', she may unintentionally upset patients with a display of her own instability.

Non-Critical Attitude: Criticism need not be by word of mouth to cause damage. A look of disdain, a shrug, a lifting of eyebrows speak for themselves.

Poise: is the state of being well-balanced. Probably one of the most difficult virtues to acquire, for it is rooted in experience, knowledge and self-confidence.

Confidence: Translated from 'con' and 'fidio' meaning 'trust'. A nurse can help the patient to have confidence in the hospital, doctors and therapies by her own belief in them. She should try to make her patient feel that health, mental and physical, is a tremendously satisfying goal to win against the odds of illness.

Listening: Eager or interested listening pays an indirect compliment to the person speaking.

Other points in the nursing of the mentally ill patient

Attitude of Superiority

It is not wise to underestimate a sick person's intelligence. Assuming a superior air implies a disrespect for the listener's intelligence. Avoid any tendency to 'talk down' to very young, very old or foreign-born patients.

Over-rating of what patients say

Speech is part of behaviour. When a sick person pays a nurse great compliments or harangues in obscene language, this is probably only an expression of his illness. In his confusion, the patient may identify the nurse with someone he greatly loves or despises.

Stimulation of ideas of reference

Sick people may misinterpret a conversation held a little distance away from them. Patients in coma, stupor or in the throes of a seizure are not always unaware of remarks and actions taking place near them.

Intimate friendships with patients

As much as a nurse may wish to become a personal friend of a patient, she forfeits her usefulness to him in so doing. There is a certain confidence and security he can place in a nurse as long as he knows that the relationship is on a professional basis.

Unfulfilled Promises

A promise to do something should not be made unless there is every indication it will be fulfilled. If a nurse fails to fulfil a promise, she must go to the person concerned and explain the state of affairs.

Hurried Contacts

Sick people everywhere complain about the way nurses hurry through conversations and treatments. A remedy for this is to give careful thought to the day's work. Convalescent patients may be given minor jobs to do, leaving the nurse more time for those who need more care and attention. Especially in this work, nurses must be prepared to sit and listen to a patient when he feels inclined to talk.

Importance of a Satisfactory Rapport

This is a must before you can attempt to carry out satisfactory psychiatric nursing care. Having built up a good relationship, you will find that the patient will respond to your care and this will help a great deal in his eventual recovery.

Practice Questions

1. What kind of foodstuffs must not be taken in conjunction with Mono-amine oxidase inhibitors (M.A.O.I.s)?
2. What part did Cerletti and Bini play in the treatment of the mentally ill?
3. Depressed patients should be encouraged to attend dances, discos, parties and other cheerful events. True?
4. What is a systematised delusion?
5. In administering E.C.T., why is the muscle relaxant given *after* the patient has been anaesthetised?

Discussion Questions

a   One of a nurse's most prized possessions is her 'licence to touch'. Why is this so?

b   Why do we make such strenuous efforts to keep the patient out of psychiatric hospitals?

c   Discuss the advantages and disadvantages of nursing staff using each other's first names, and encouraging patients to do so too. Could this be done in general hospitals?

d   Virtually every psychiatric hospital has more female residents than male. Why is this so?

e   In certain cases it may be said that some patients suffer from 'an insufficiency of neglect'. When might this be true?

f   'Uniforms act as a barrier between nurses and patients'. Is this a reasonable statement?

g   There is a difference between 'nursing care' and 'nursing actions'. What is it?

Answers
1. Foods containing Tyramine, e.g. cheese, Bovril, Marmite, broad beans.
2. Cerletti and Bini developed electroplexy (E.C.T.) from work done by von Meduna earlier.
3. It is generally true that patients suffering from exogenous (reactive, neurotic) depression will benefit from attending cheerful functions. The patient suffering from endogenous (psychotic) depression may not; being forced to participate in social activities may worsen his condition. Many 'normal' people greatly dislike such activities. Psychiatric illness rarely changes this state of affairs, and their wishes must be respected. Having said this, many patients are merely apathetic and decline social activity, but find that they enjoy themselves once they become involved.
4. A systematised delusion is one which is complex. Events are arranged in the patient's mind to substantiate his beliefs.
5. Muscle relaxants are given *after* the anaesthetic, since to a conscious patient the experience of feeling unable to move, and unable to breathe, would be very traumatic and, indeed, unbearable. Hence, in surgery, as in E.C.T., the patient is totally anaesthetised first.

10 LEGAL ASPECTS OF PSYCHIATRY

The Mental Health Act (1983)

Legislation for the mentally disordered has often proved the source of prolonged and often bitter debate between interested parties.

Since the first major piece of legislation appeared in the form of the monumental 'Lunacy Act' of 1890, legislation has sought to reflect the changing social attitudes towards the mentally ill, and the increasing knowledge regarding the causation and treatments of many mental disorders.

The enlightened, some would claim, revolutionary, Mental Health Act of 1959, did much to reflect the growing trend in acceptance of the mentally disordered and to attempt to break down the barriers between physical and mental illness.

Since then, many changes have occurred and these are once more reflected in the present Mental Health Act of 1983, which came into force on 30 September 1983.

In the table following, extracts provide a mere outline of some of the main provisions of the Act. Readers are urged to increase the depth of their knowledge by consulting the Act itself, or any of the numerous textbooks that are available on the subject.

The Mental Health Act, 1983 is divided into several parts, each dealing with specific areas of conduct towards the mentally disordered, and the technical provisions required by the Act.

Below are printed several terms which appear elsewhere in the text. They are explained so that the reader will find it easier to understand the functions of each in the context of implementation of the Act.

Mental Health Act Commission

The Mental Health Act, 1983, provides for a Commission with special functions. The Commission consists of 80 members, appointed by the Secretary of State and drawn from the disciplines of Psychiatry, Law, Psychology, Social Work, and so on.

The chief responsibilities of the Commission include:

1. Monitoring the execution of the Act.
2. To appoint 'second independent opinions' from doctors and other appropriate disciplines.
3. To monitor the care and welfare of individual patients (initially, concern will be with 'detained' patients).
4. The inspection of hospitals.
5. To inspect, where necessary, any records relating to the treatment of any past or present patients in particular hospitals visited.

Mental Health Review Tribunal

The Mental Health Review Tribunals are concerned with applications from certain detained patients (or, in some cases, their relatives), who feel that they have been wrongfully detained in hospital.

The Tribunal consists of at least three members, drawn from the disciplines of Law, Psychiatry and 'Lay' persons (often with some experience of Social Administration).

Among the main functions of the Tribunals are the following:
1. Directing the discharge of a patient.
2. Directing the discharge of a patient at a future date.
3. Recommending that the patient be granted leave of absence.
4. Recommending transfer to another hospital or into guardianship.

Approved Social Worker

Local Authorities are empowered by the Act to appoint sufficient numbers of Approved Social Workers in order to carry out certain requirements of the Act.

No Social Worker shall be 'Approved' unless he is considered by the Authority as having the appropriate competence in dealing with persons suffering from mental disorder.

Information to Detained Patients

The Act required that the managers of the hospital or mental nursing home in which a patient is legally detained, shall take such steps as is practicable to ensure that the patient understands:
1. Under which provisions of the Act he is being detained.
2. What rights exist for applying to a Mental Health Tribunal regarding his detention.
The information must be given orally and in writing (Hospitals have printed forms with the relevant information already set out in detail.)

A copy of the information given is forwarded to the nearest relative (unless the patient requests otherwise).

Individuals may enter hospital without legal formality, i.e. the individual in need of care and treatment may agree voluntarily to be admitted to hospital. 'Informal' patients constitute by far the largest number of patients within psychiatric hospitals.

A minority of patients who, for a variety of reasons, may refuse to enter hospital voluntarily, but are nevertheless in need of psychiatric care and treatment, may be admitted to hospital 'formally', i.e. under certain legal provisions contained in the Mental Health Act, 1983. They are then said to be compulsorily detained.

Still other patients, again in the minority, may, through their involvement in certain criminal proceedings, be referred for admission to hospital by a Magistrate or Crown Court. Once more, the Mental Health Act, 1983, makes provision for this.

Patients who are compulsorily detained are admitted on certain 'Sections' of the Act.

The following chart outlines several of the main 'Sections' commonly applied.

N.B.   Because of the complexity of the 'Sections' which refer to patients who are admitted by direction of a Court of Law because of their involvement in criminal proceedings, they do not appear in this text. Readers are advised to consult the Act itself, or any of the numerous specialist textbooks which are available.

For those that consult the Act, the relevant 'Sections' referred to are to be found in Part III of the Act — Sections 35 to 55).

Section 1

Definition of Mental Disorder
Under the Act, the term 'Mental Disorder' is defined as follows.

1. Mental Illness
Not further defined, but includes the chief categories of mental illness, namely the psychoses and the neuroses.

2. Mental Impairment
Means a state of arrested or incomplete development of mind which includes significant impairment of intelligence and social functioning and is associated with abnormally aggressive or seriously irresponsible conduct on the part of the person concerned.

3. Severe Mental Impairment

Means a state of arrested or incomplete development of mind which includes severe mental impairment of intelligence and social functioning and is associated with abnormally aggressive or seriously irresponsible conduct on the part of the person concerned.

4. Psychopathic Disorder

Means a persistent disorder or disability of mind (whether or not including significant impairment of intelligence), which results in abnormally aggressive or seriously irresponsible behaviour on the part of the person concerned.

5. Any Other Disorder or Disability of Mind

(A person may not be regarded as suffering from mental disorder by reason of promiscuity, or other immoral conduct; sexual deviancy; dependence on alcohol/drugs, alone).

Consent to Treatment

The provisions of the Act regarding treatment of patients are very detailed and intricate. Because of this, only the briefest details are set out below.

For a more detailed account, readers are advised to refer to the appropriate part of the Act itself, or to other, more informative references in other textbooks.

(If the Act is consulted, the relevant Sections are 56 to 64).

Section 57

Treatment requiring consent **and** a second opinion.

This section deals with the administration of certain potentially hazardous/dangerous treatments, which include:
1. Any surgical operation for destroying brain tissue.
2. Any other form of treatment that may be specified by the Secretary of State in regulations.

Before Treatment can be given

a The patient (either *'informally'* or *'formally'* detained). **Must** give consent to the treatment being carried out.
   and
b An independent doctor, and two other persons, appointed by the M.H.A. Commission, have certified in writing that the patient is capable of understanding the nature, purpose and likely effects of the proposed treatment — and has consented to it.

c The independent doctor has certified in writing that the treatment is the appropriate one under the circumstances. (Having first consulted with **two** other persons who have professional involvement with the patient's treatment — one of whom must be a nurse, the other either a nurse or a doctor).

Section 58
Treatment requiring consent **or** a second opinion.

This Section refers to the administration of medicines (by any means) and such treatments specified by the Secretary of State in regulations (which includes E.C.T.).

No detained patient may be given E.C.T. or medicines after the first **three months** unless:
1. The patient has given consent which has been certified by either the Responsible Medical Officer **or** an independent doctor.
2. An independent doctor has certified in writing that the patient is not capable of understanding the nature, purpose and likely effects of the treatment, or has not given consent. The independent doctor certifies that continuing with the treatment will be likely to alleviate or prevent deterioration of the patient's condition. The patient should, therefore, continue to receive treatment, even without consent being given.

Section 62
Urgent treatment
Under certain conditions, a **detained patient** may be given treatment without formally consenting or without the need for a 'second independent opinion'.

Treatment may be given if:
1. It is immediately necessary to save the life of the patient.
2. It is immediately necessary to prevent a serious deterioration of the patient's condition (this **excludes** 'irreversible treatment').
3. It is immediately necessary and is the minimum necessary to prevent the patient from behaving violently or being a danger to himself or other (this **excludes** 'irreversible' and 'hazardous' treatments).

N.B.
'Irreversible treatment' refers to treatments which have unfavourable, irreversible physical or psychological consequences.

'Hazardous treatments' are treatments which involve potentially significant physical hazards.

TITLE OF SECTION	REASONS FOR IMPLEMENTA-TION OF THE SECTION	APPLICATION FOR COMPULSORY ADMISSION TO HOSPITAL MADE BY:	NUMBER OF MEDICAL RECOMMEN-DATIONS REQUIRED	DURATION OF SECTION	RIGHTS OF APPEAL TO THE MENTAL HEALTH REVIEW TRIBUNAL	REMARKS
Section 2 Admission for assessment or for assessment followed by medical treatment.	Persons suffering from any form of mental disorder, the degree of which warrants detention in hospital and is in the interests of their own health and safety or the protection of others.	1. Nearest Relative **OR** 2. Approved Social Worker	**TWO** are required (**ONE** must be an 'approved' Doctor)	28 days	Patient may apply within the first 14 days of admission.	
Section 3 Admission for treatment.	As above	As above	**TWO** are required	6 months	1. Patient can apply at any time within the 6 months. 2. Nearest relative can apply on behalf of the patient within 28 days.	After the first 6 months, a further period of 6 months may be applied for by the Doctor in charge of the patient. Thereafter, the Section may be extended for periods of ONE year.

Section	Conditions	Application	Medical recommendation	Duration	Appeal	Notes
Section 4 Admission for assessment in an emergency.	As above	As above	**ONE** is required (Preferably one acquainted with the patient. Often, the patient's G.P. is involved).	72 hours	An appeal is not allowed.	Upon expiry of the Section, the patient must be allowed to leave hospital if he so wishes, unless further powers have been taken to detain the patient under Section 2 and 3.
Section 5 (2) Application in respect of a patient already receiving treatment in hospital on an 'Informal' basis.	As above Additionally, the 'Holding Power' must not be enforced until all other methods of persuading the patient to stay have been used.	1. Doctor in charge of the patient's treatment. **OR** 2. His nominated deputy.	**ONE** is required	72 hours	An Appeal is not allowed.	Upon expiry, as Section 4 above.
Section 5 (4) Nurse Holding Power. (In respect of a patient already receiving treatment in hospital on an 'Informal' basis.)	The Section is to be enforced because it is not immediately practicable to secure the attendance of registered Medical Practitioner to furnish an application under Section 5 (2).	Nurse of the 'Prescribed Class' (i.e. R.M.N., R.N.M.S.).	**None** required	Up to 6 hours	An appeal is not allowed.	If the patient when eventually interviewed by the Medical Practitioner, is considered to warrant further detention under Section 5 (2), the total amount of time spent under Section 5 (4) is deducted from the 72 hours required by Section 5 (2).

Avenues of Discharge

Patients in hospital can be discharged in the following ways:

1. **'Informal' patients:**
   Patients who have entered hospital without legal formality are technically free to leave hospital whenever they so choose.

2. **'Formally Detained' patients**
   Patients who are legally detained in hospital can be discharged via a variety of mechanisms, depending upon the nature of their detention, and the legal requirements of the 'Section' under which they are detained.

   The avenues of discharge may include:
   1. When the Responsible Medical Officer deems appropriate.
   2. On expiry of a 'Section', when no further powers are taken to extend or convert a Section to another.
   3. At the request of the Hospital Managers.
   4. At the direction of the Mental Health Review Tribunal (Where appropriate).
   5. By 'process of law', i.e. if a patient detained under certain Sections of the Act, is absent without leave from the hospital for a designated amount of time, without being detected.
   6. At the request of the nearest relative, giving 72 hours notice, in writing, of the intention to discharge a relative.

Practice Questions

Mark the following statements True or False
1. Section 2 is for admission for assessment or for assessment and treatment.
2. Section 5 (4) provides for a doctor to detain a patient already in hospital on an 'Informal' basis.
3. The Mental Health Act, 1983, came into force on 30 August, 1983.
4. Social Workers will need to be approved by Local Authorities.
5. Persons detained in hospital under Section 4 of the Act, can appeal to a Mental Health Review Tribunal.
6. Only one medical recommendation is required to detain a patient on Section 2 of the Act.
7. Section 3 of the Act is for 6 months duration.
8. A patient who suffers from mental impairment cannot be detained in hospital under Section 1 of the Act.
9. A patient who requires to be admitted to hospital compulsorily under Section 4 of the Act, must have been seen by the applicant within 24 hours previously.

10. Section 57 of the Act provides for compulsory treatment which requires patient consent or a second opinion.
11. A patient cannot be detained under the Act unless he/she has achieved the age of 14 years.
12. The nearest relative can apply to discharge a detained relative from hospital if he/she is detained under Section 2 of the Act.
13. The nurse 'Holding Power' of 6 hours, and portions of this time limit, form part of an eventual 72 hour period of Section 5 (2).
14. A person detained in hospital on Section 3 of the Act, has more opportunities to apply to a Mental Health Review Tribunal.
15. Section 3 of the Act lasts for 6 months.
16. Social Workers will need to be 'approved' by October, 1984.
17. No detained patient can be given medicines without consent or a second medical opinion after four months have lapsed since first administration.
18. Section 136 involves a police constable removing an apparently mentally disordered person from a public place to a place of safety.
19. Under the new Act, 'Mental Disorder' is defined as:-
Mental Illness/ Mental Impairment/ Severe Mental Impairment/ Psychopathic Disorder.
20. The new Mental Health Commission has the power to inspect hospitals for the treatment and care of the mentally ill and mentally impaired.

Answers

 1. True
 2. False
 3. False
 4. True
 5. False
 6. False
 7. True
 8. True
 9. True
10. False
11. True
12. True
13. True
14. False
15. True
16. True
17. False
18. True
19. True
20. True

11 GLOSSARY OF PSYCHOLOGICAL AND PSYCHIATRIC TERMS

Abreaction
An emotional release or discharge that results from mentally reliving or recalling to awareness a painful experience which has been forgotten (repressed) because it was intolerable to conscious awareness.
The therapeutic effect of abreaction is through the discharge of painful emotions, thereby relieving the person of their influence.

Affect
A generalized feeling distinguished from emotion in being more persistent and pervasive.
The sum of reactions arising in connection with an emotion. It may be regarded as having quantitative attributes capable of increase, diminution, displacement, and elimination. Used synonymously with **mood**.

Aggression
A feeling or action that is hostile or self-assertive.

Ambivalence
Opposing emotions, desires or attitudes existing at the same time toward an object or person. Ambivalent feelings may be conscious, partly hidden from conscious awareness or one aspect of the feelings may be unconscious, e.g. the coexistence of love and hate toward the same person.

Amnesia
A pathological loss of memory which may vary in length of time or degree of loss. It may be psychological, organic or of mixed origin.

Anxiety
A state of apprehensive tension or uneasiness which stems from the imminent anticipation of danger when the source is largely unknown or unrecognised.

Apathy
A state of absence of emotions: a want of feeling, or lack of emotion.

Attitude
An attitude is a predisposition to respond in a persistent and characteristic manner, usually positively or negatively (for or against), in reference to some situation, material, object, or class of objects, or person or group of persons. Attitudes are always learned, not inborn.

Autism: Autistic thinking
A form of thinking which is highly subjective and is essentially non-conforming to that generally common to society; it gratifies unfulfilled personal desires without the regard for the demands of reality; more or less equivalent to wishful thinking, or fantasy and day dreaming.

Aura
Subjective feelings preceding an epileptic seizure.

Automatism
Automatic, mechanical and apparently undirected symbolic behaviour which is outside conscious control.

Behaviour
The total response, motor and glandular, which an organism makes to any situation with which it is faced.

Belief
An attitude involving the recognition or acceptance of something as factual, and not necessarily supported by reason.

Catalepsy
A condition of stupor with muscular rigidity and sustained immobility.

Character
This is the mental and moral equipment acquired from education and the environment and is revealed in the conduct of the individual and his relations with other people.

Chorea
Motor disorder characterised by involuntary, jerky, spasmodic movements.

Clonic
Refers to rapid contraction and relaxation of antagonistic groups of muscles.

Coma
A state of deep unconsciousness with non-responsiveness to stimulation.

Compulsion
An insistent, repetitive, intensive and unwanted urge to perform an act which is contrary to the patient's ordinary conscious wishes or standards. A compulsion is a defensive substitute for hidden and still more unacceptable ideas and wishes.

Conation
Pertaining to the basic strivings of the individual, as expressed in his behaviour and actions.

Conditioning
This is a process of learning in which a new way of reacting to a situation is developed. It occurs when there is added temporarily to the situation a stimulus that is sufficient to produce a different reaction.

Confabulation
The filling in of memory gaps with made-up episodes.

Conflict
The clash between two opposing emotional forces which may be conscious or unconscious. A painful state of consciousness resulting from the existence of opposing desires, emotions or goals.

Confusion
Disturbed orientation in respect of time, place or person, which is sometimes accompanied by disturbances of consciousness.

Conscience
An individual's system of accepted moral principles or principles of conduct.

Consciousness
The mental state of awareness (alertness) which maintains an interpretations contact of the individual with the environment both internal and external.

Constitution
The total inherent physical and mental endowment of a person.

Conversion
The process by which an emotional conflict is expressed as a physical symptom.

Culture
The social organization characteristic of a particular group of people.

Cyclothymia
Describes a tendency to alternating excitement and depression.

Déjà Vu
The subjective feeling that an experience which is occurring for the first time has happened before.

Delirium
A state of mental disturbance characterized by confusion, disordered speech and often by hallucination.

Delirium Tremens
An acute frightening delirium occurring in severe chronic alcoholism upon withdrawal of alcohol.

Delusion
A false belief not in harmony with the individual's race, creed or education, which cannot be corrected by an appeal to logic or reason.

Dementia
A deterioration of intellectual powers, generally owing to organic or functional disorders.

Depersonalization
Loss of the sense of personal identity and feelings of unreality or strangeness — a feeling of being someone else or something else.

Disorientation
This is the loss, sometimes temporarily, by an individual of his perception of his relationship with regard to space, time or persons.

Displacement
A mechanism whereby the emotions associated with one idea or object are unconsiously attached to another.

Disposition
Man's disposition describes the totality of natural tendencies to act in certain ways — usually with emphasis on the effective and impulsive aspects.

Dissociation
A disorder of the mental system in which one or two groups of ideas become split off from the main body of the personality and are not accessible to consciousness.

Distractibility
A disorder of thought and speech in which attention is unduly distracted by the environment or by the patient's psychic dissociation.

Echolalia
Involuntary and meaningless repetition of words heard spoken by others; a symptom of schizophrenia.

Echopraxia
Involuntary and meaningless repetition of gestures or movements made by others — a symptom of schizophrenia.

Ego
The conscious self; that part of the mind which develops to deal with reality.

Emotion
A distinctive feeling tone, such as love, hate, fear, etc. It may be described as a complex state of the organism, involving bodily changes of a widespread character — in breathing, pulse, gland secretion etc. — and on the mental side, a state of excitement or perturbation marked by strong feeling and usually an impulse towards a definite form of behaviour.

Empathy
The capacity of feeling in communication with others.

Epilepsy
May be defined as a sudden transient disturbance of cerebral function which, if it is sufficiently widespread, involves loss of consciousness and in certain forms convulsive seizures.

Euphoria
An exaggerated sense of well-being.

Extraversion
The direction of interest and emotions toward the environment.

Fantasy
An imaginary sequence of events of mental images.

Fixation
Arrest of an emotional progression at some intermediate stage of development.

Flexibilitas Cerea
Waxy flexibility: Cataleptic state in which limbs remain in any position in which they may be placed — a symptom of some types of schizophrenia.

Flight of ideas
Rapid succession of superficially related or entirely unrelated ideas producing such digressions as to prevent reaching the goal idea of a narrative, occurring in manic states.

Folie á Deux
A delusion or delusional system shared by two individuals, usually a husband and wife, or two sisters.

Fugue
A major state of personality dissociation characterized by loss of memory.

Furor
Acute emotional excitement involving violent behaviour.

Globus Hystericus
A choking sensation as though a ball were in the throat: hysterical spasm of the oesophagus.

Grandiose
That which is characterized by affectation, eminence, magnificence or splendour.

Group Test
An intelligence, achievement, personality or aptitude test applied to a number of persons at one time in which responses are written.

Habit
A habit is a learned, mechanized behaviour pattern or way of doing something.

Hallucination
This is an experience having the character of sense perception, but without relevant or adequate sensory stimulus, i.e. an imaginary sense perception. The patient will insist he hears voices, sees persons or objects etc., when actually there is no external stimulus for such assertions.

Hallucinosis
Disordered mental condition subject to the occurrence of hallucinations, without any other necessary impairment of consciousness.

Heterosexual
Sexual attraction for or towards persons of the opposite sex.

Homosexual
Sexual attraction for or towards a person of the same sex.

Hypnosis
An altered state of conscious awareness which is induced in a cooperative subject.

Id
A psychoanalytical term used to denote the unconscious part of the personality which contains primitive urges and desires and is ruled by the pleasure principle.

Ideas of reference
The incorrect interpretation by an individual of casual incidents and external events as having some direct reference to himself.

Identification
A mental mechanism by which one feels or thinks as another person.
A mental mechanism operating outside of and beyond conscious awareness by which an individual endeavours to make himself resemble another.

Illusion
The misinterpretation of a real, external, sensory experience, e.g. the patient insists a grey sock on the floor is a mouse.

Insight
A reasonably accurate self-judgement including the emotional acceptance of one's self.

Instinct
An instinct is an innate determining tendency. It should be noted that an instinct is not a form of behaviour, but rather an underlying impulse, more or less equivalent to a 'drive' or 'need'.

Intellect
Mind in its cognitive aspect, and particularly with reference to the higher thought processes.

Intelligence
Intelligence is innate, general, mental energy capable of being transferred to any activity.
Intelligence is the capacity to meet novel situations, or learn to do so, by new adaptive responses.
Intelligence is the ability to perform tests or tasks involving the grasping of relationships, the degree of intelligence being proportional to the complexity and the abstraction, or both of the relationships.

Intelligence quotient
This is the ratio of mental age to chronological age expressed as a percentage.

Introversion
The direction of interests and emotions towards oneself.

Jacksonian epilepsy
Form of epilepsy with localized spasms in one limb, or on one side of the body, and usually without loss of consciousness; taken as indicating irritation in motor zones or cortex.

Korsakoffs syndrome
A mental disorder, or group of symptoms, caused by disordered metabolism, usually from chronic alcoholism, and characterized by memory, orientation, and retention defects and confabulation; polyneuritis often accompanies it.

Learning
Learning is the modification and control of behaviour so as to make it more effective and better adapted to the situation present.
Learning is the process of organizing experience by discovering and developing meaningful relations.

Libido
A psychosomatic (Freudian) term meaning, the vital force or psychic energy which motivates living.
A term often used to imply 'sex drive'.

Memory
Memory is the full, accurate recall of the required material at the required time.
Memory is that characteristic of living organisms in virtue of which what they experience leaves behind effects which modify future experience and behaviour.

Mental mechanisms
These are unconscious processes of the mind whereby conflict is evaded or made less painful when it cannot be solved at the rational level.
Psychological methods of thinking or acting which serve to solve conflicts and meet the needs of the personality.

Milieu
The immediate environment, physical and social, but usually, in psychology, with emphasis on the latter.

Mood
Moods are affective experiences which last longer and are less intense than emotions.

Motive
Motives are a source of driving power from within, producing behaviour.

Need
A condition marked by the feeling of lack or want of something, or requiring the performance of some action.
Negativism
A generalized resistance to any suggestion from outside the self.
Neologism
The invention of new words: usually coined by condensation of other words.
Word symbol seen particularly in schizophrenia.

Obsession
The uncontrollable urge to concentrate upon some thought or to perform some obviously unnecessary action.
Overcompensation
An exaggerated attempt to make up for a known defect, the attempt being determined sometimes by the unconscious.

Perception
Perception is understanding by the mind through any of the six senses.
Personality
The integrated and dynamic organization of the individual, as that manifests itself to other people in the give and take of social life.
Personality is the aggregate of the physical, mental, emotional, social, moral and spiritual characteristics of the individual.
Personality is the organization of the sum total of the behaviour patterns of the individual.
Persuasion
The process of influencing, or seeking to influence, an individual's opinions and actions, ostensibly by reasoning or intellectual appeal though depending for its effectiveness in most cases on non-rational factors.
Phobia
A compulsive fear or a morbid fear, of an object, situation or act.
Pleasure principle
The regulation of activity with the purpose of avoiding pain or procuring pleasure.
Preconscious
Not present in consciousness at a given moment, but recallable more or less readily when wanted.
Prejudice
An attitude, usually with an emotional colouring hostile to, or in favour of, action or objects of a certain kind, certain persons, and certain doctrines.

Projection
A mental mechanism in which perceptions, motives, desires thoughts and activities, stemming from within the self, are attributed to the external environment.

Psychoanalysis
A system of psychology, elaborated by Sigmund Freud, and a method of treatment of mental illness, characterized by a dynamic view of all aspects of the mental life, conscious and unconscious, with special emphasis on the phenomena of the unconscious and by an elaborate technique of investigation and treatment, based on the employment of conscious free association.

Rapport
Relations which are characterized by harmony, conformity and accord. Confidence of the patient in the psychotherapist.

Rationalizaton
This is the mechanism whereby guilty or culpable behaviour is justified at any cost, though the individual is unaware of what he is doing.
A mental mechanism whereby the patient substitutes a plausible reason for the real one motivating his behaviour.

Reality principle
The regulation of activity in accordance with the demands of reality.

Regression
A mental mechanism whereby an individual reverts to patterns of behaviour characteristic of an earlier phase of development.

Repression
A mental mechanism which operates unconsciously to keep from awareness unpleasant experiences, emotions and ideas. The repressed material is submerged into unconsciousness, but remains dynamic.

Retardation
Pathological slowness or delay of mental and motor responses.

Rote learning
Learning by pure repetition, regardless of meaning, and without any attempt at organization.

Schizoid
A personality type, tending towards dissociation of the emotional from the intellectual life; a shut-in personality.
Resembling schizophrenia; term applied to personalities that are predominantly introverted.

Senility
The impairment, particularly of mental functions, present in old age.

Socialization
The process by which the individual is adapted to his social en-

vironment, and becomes a recognized cooperating and efficient member of it.

Stereotypy

A pathological symptom showing itself in continuous repetition of seemingly senseless words and syllables, or to certain postures and actions.

Stupor

Reduced responsiveness; partial or complete unconsciousness. Present in catatonia, depression and hysteria.

Subconscious

That part of the mind which is not focused in awareness, but which is capable of affecting conscious mental or physical reactions.

Sublimation

Defined as 'biologically and socially useful re-directions of emotional energy'.

A mental mechanism whereby the energy associated with primitive drives is successfully utilized in constructive social activities.

Suggestibility

Readiness to accept suggestion, as a temporary or permanent characteristic of the individual.

Suggestion

Suggestion is all the processes by which one mind acts on, or is acted on, by another unwittingly.

Suggestion is the process of communication resulting in the acceptance with conviction of the communicated proposition, in the absence of logically adequate grounds for its acceptance.

Super-ego

A psychoanalytic term used to describe the critical aspect of the personality which is usually equated with the popular term conscience.

A term used to designate a structure in the unconscious built up by early experiences, on the basis mainly of the child's relations to his parents, and functioning as a kind of conscience, criticizing the thoughts and acts of the ego, causing feelings of guilt and anxiety, when the ego gratifies or tends to gratify primitive impulses.

Suppression

Suppression is the deliberate, conscious, willed rejection of an impulse in the interest of self control or some other higher value.

A mental mechanism whereby unpleasant feelings and experiences are deliberately kept from awareness.

Symbol

An object or activity representing, and standing as a substitute for, something else; in psychoanalytical theory, a representation by something not directly connected with it, of unconscious, usually repressed sexual material.

Symbolization
The process of employing symbols in dreams, myths and the like; characteristically present also in neurotic symptoms.

Temperament
Temperament is the personal qualities determined by the chemical influence of the body metabolism, exerted on the brain and nervous system.
Temperament is the particular mode in which the emotions are felt by different minds; the mode in which the emotions are manifested.

Tension
A feeling of strain; a general sense of disturbance of equilibrium, and of readiness to alter behaviour to meet some almost threatening factor in the situation.

Tic
An intermittent spasmodic or jerky movement (generally one of the head or face muscles), as a rule originating in some neurotic disturbance.

Tonic
A muscular spasm characterized by tonicity or sustained contraction, such as is observed during the 'stiffening' phase of a convulsion.

Trait
An individual characteristic in thought, feeling, or act, inherited or acquired.

Transference
The unconscious identification of another person in a role with which an individual has had past experience.
The Freudian concept of the emotional situation which develops between patient and psychiatrist, wherein the patient transfers either affection or hostility to the physician. The attitude is transient and unconscious.

Twilight states
A rare condition marked by a peculiar alteration of consciousness and personality for a certain period of time of limited duration, with subsequent amnesia.

Unconscious
That part of mental activity which is not accessible to conscious awareness.

Volition
The conscious adoption by the individual of a line of action.
Self conscious activity towards a determined end, manifested primarily in decision and intention.

12   ADVICE FOR EXAMINATION PREPARATION

Start your preparation well in advance of the examination. Make a realistic plan of action that you will be able to achieve.
1. Decide how many hours each day you can set aside for study/revision 2 hours daily × 5 = 10 hours weekly.
2. Make a timetable and slot in all the subjects to be studied. The length of time you allocate depends on the level of difficulty.
3. Study in the same place each day. Sit at a desk or table and have the materials you need at hand, i.e. paper, pencils, crayons, text books, lecture notes and a rubber. Write in pencil so that mistakes or unwanted notes can be erased (paper is expensive).
4. You must work at concentrating on your task, don't allow yourself to think of anything else so that you waste time.
5. If you are tired or upset, relax before attempting to settle.
6. Work at each of the goals you have set yourself as widely as you can.
7. Reward yourself when a goal is achieved so that you associate pleasure with studying.
8. Success is not a matter of luck but of good planning and self-discipline.
9. Learning is an active process so:
   a   Study using a logical approach. Sequence the material and go from easy to more difficult concepts.
   b   Don't try to learn chunks of material, skim the passage and try to understand. Underline key words or sentences. Use a dictionary.
   c   Overlearn material and consciously recall and reinforce your memory. Commit your thoughts to paper.
   d   Use mnemonics as a memory aid.
   e   Ask yourself questions, apply the material, compare with management of actual patients you have nursed. Have discussions with friends/tutors.
   f   Ask your tutors for help if you do not understand the relevance of a topic.
   g   Learn to draw and label line drawings correctly.
   h   Test yourself using past examination questions.
   i   Get your relations or friends to ask you questions.

10. Cultivate a fast reading style. Use several textbooks with your notes. Make your own notes when you have analysed the meaning of a passage. Begin to read with a question in mind and ask yourself questions when you have read a paragraph/chapter. Read quickly then re-read.

11. What you want to achieve is efficiency of study with economy of effort.

Examination technique

1. Listen to the invigilator's instructions and follow them carefully. Have your number card signed and available for inspection. Be prepared with pens, pencils, a rubber and ruler.

2. Read the instructions on the front cover of the book and comply with them, i.e. start a question on a fresh page, number your questions carefully, write legibly. Note how many questions are to be attempted, how much time is allowed etc.

3. Objective type questions test a wide area of knowledge, recognition and recall in a short time. Consider the questions carefully, and choose what you believe to be the correct answer from the distractors, do not just guess.

4. Essay questions test:
   a Knowledge
   b Comprehension
   c Application
   d Communication
   e Synthesis

5. Read all the questions carefully on both sides of the paper, identify all parts of the question.
   a Don't be concerned that others have started to write.
   b Select the questions you feel most able to answer.
   c Tick your selection in order of sequence.
   d Analyse the setting of the question. Is the scene in hospital or the community? What is the importance of age, sex, marital/ social status, environment, psychological well-being, needs of the patient in the examiner's mind.
      Underline these points and develop them.
   e Note the essential points that have to be made in your answer in the margin of the paper.
   f Pay attention to the weighting of each part of the question, these should help you plan the time to be spent on each part.
   g Ten minutes spent in planning is the most effective way of using the examination time.
   h When you start to write:

  (i)   answer the parts in order of a, b, c, d.
 (ii)   write legibly, be logical (first things first)
(iii)   concentrate on the main parts, don't waffle and repeat yourself.
(iv)   if a diagram is asked for make a clear line drawing and label it clearly.
 (v)   leave time at the end for reading your answers.

Remember that a good essay has an introduction, a development and a conclusion, and should be clear and concise.

NOTES